Breathe Easy

Donald A. Mahler, MD

Breathe Easy

Relieving the Symptoms of Chronic Lung Disease

(ForeEdge)

ForeEdge

An imprint of University Press of New England

www.upne.com

© 2017 University Press of New England

All rights reserved

Manufactured in the United States of America

Designed by Eric M. Brooks

Typeset in Arnhem by Passumpsic Publishing

Library of Congress Cataloging-in-Publication Data

NAMES: Mahler, Donald A., author.

TITLE: Breathe easy: relieving the symptoms of chronic lung
    disease / Donald A. Mahler, MD.

DESCRIPTION: Lebanon, NH: ForeEdge, [2017] |
    Includes bibliographical references and index.

IDENTIFIERS: LCCN 2016056078 (print) | LCCN 2017001996
    (ebook) | ISBN 9781611689013 (cloth) | ISBN 9781611689020
    (pbk.) | ISBN 9781512600803 (epub, mobi & pdf)

SUBJECTS: LCSH: Lungs—Diseases. | Lungs—Diseases—
    Treatment.

CLASSIFICATION: LCC RC756 .M24 2017 (print) |
    LCC RC756 (ebook) | DDC 616.2/4—dc23

LC record available at https://lccn.loc.gov/2016056078

5 4 3 2 1

For my grandchildren

Emma Layne Richardson

Jack Mahler Richardson

Ella Claire Colgan &

Bennett Donald Morrison

You are my inspiration

Contents

Preface

Another glorious day, the air as delicious to the lungs
as nectar to the tongue.
John Muir, conservationist (1838–1914)

Breathe Easy aims to educate and to help those who experience breathing difficulty. Most people don't think about breathing because it is an automatic and unconscious act. However, the majority of those with asthma (twenty-five million Americans), chronic obstructive pulmonary disease (twenty-four million Americans), and interstitial lung disease (one to two million Americans) become aware of their shortness of breath when it interferes with work and daily activities. A former tagline of the American Lung Association describes what anyone who has a breathing problem knows quite well: "When you can't breathe, nothing else matters." As a result, individuals seek medical care to find out why they are short of breath and to receive treatment in order to *Breathe Easy*.

Before writing this book, I searched Amazon for books about "breathing" that were written for the public. The following three books were listed:

1 *Breathe Free: Nutritional and Herbal Care for Your Respiratory System* (1990)
2 *The Breathing Book: Good Health and Vitality through Essential Breath Work* (1996)
3 *The Healing Power of the Breath: Simple Techniques to Reduce Stress and Anxiety, Enhance Concentration, and Balance Your Emotions* (2012)

The first two books were published more than twenty years ago. The third book concerns the emotional aspects of breathing. The paucity of books demonstrates a major gap of current information for those who experience breathing difficulty.

Breathe Easy is written to fill this gap. The book offers unique information to millions of Americans and others throughout the world who are bothered or limited by their breathing. The book addresses "key" issues faced by those who experience shortness of breath. It is intended for those who want to learn more about breathing and practical ways to make it easier. In particular, those with asthma, chronic obstructive pulmonary disease, or interstitial lung disease will benefit from reading specific chapters in the book that address these common respiratory diseases. Family members and caregivers will also be interested as they often ask, "What can I do to help?" The contents of this book provide helpful information.

The initial chapter describes how to breathe. This basic information is important for understanding the experience of breathing difficulty. The next chapter reviews "second wind," a phrase commonly used to describe renewed energy or effort. The five common causes of chronic shortness of breath—anemia, anxiety, deconditioning, heart disease, and lung disease—are considered in the third chapter. This information helps the reader understand the challenges of the health-care provider to find the correct diagnosis. After chapters on asthma and chronic obstructive pulmonary disease, the correct use of inhalers is discussed and illustrated. This information is critical for inhaling medications deep into the lungs to achieve the greatest effect. Then, important information about interstitial lung disease, the third most common chronic respiratory disease, is reviewed. In chapter 8, the effects of aging on the brain and on the body are presented, followed by consideration of the overall benefits of exercise. The penultimate chapter describes other strategies that can be tried to relieve shortness of breath. A final chapter offers unique information about traveling with oxygen.

From my biased perspective, this book is "one of a kind" for anyone and everyone who experiences breathing difficulty. It is informative and a practical guide to better breathing. I wish all of you the ability to *Breathe Easy*.

Donald A. Mahler, MD

Acknowledgments

All chapters in *Breathe Easy* have been revised multiple times after review and comments by several individuals. I am grateful for the insights provided by Susan McNeely and Carl Small based on their perspectives and personal experiences. Special thanks to Alex H. Gifford, MD, assistant professor of medicine at Geisel School of Medicine at Dartmouth; Scott Astle, RRT, and clinical coordinator of cardiorespiratory services at Valley Regional Hospital in Claremont, New Hampshire; Mary Anne Riley, RRT, and program coordinator of pulmonary rehabilitation programs at Springfield Hospital in Springfield, Vermont, and at Cheshire Medical Center in Keene, New Hampshire; and Drew Carter, senior sales representative—respiratory for Lincare Inc., in Enfield, New Hampshire.

I appreciate the creative efforts of Kyle Morrison (kyle@left rightcreative.com) who designed the figures that illustrate important concepts. The collective input from these individuals has helped to provide practical information about breathing that should positively affect the daily lives of the readers.

Breathe Easy

(1)

How to Breathe

Breathing in I calm my body. Breathing out I smile. Dwelling in
the present moment, I know this is a wonderful moment!

Thich Nhat Hanh, Vietnamese Buddhist monk and author (1926–)

Breathing is essential to life. One purpose of each and every breath
is to take in oxygen. However, it is equally important that we get rid
of carbon dioxide—a waste product of our body—during exhalation. To understand how to breathe, it is helpful to review the parts
(anatomy) and workings (function) of the respiratory system. This
information provides a framework for knowing about various lung
conditions if you, or a loved one, has a breathing problem.

How to breathe depends on the interactions between the brain
and the respiratory system. These areas are connected by nerves
(called the nervous system) that enable communication by electrical signals that travel back and forth. Sensors in the respiratory
system provide information to the brain about breathing, and the
brain controls how fast and how deep to breathe.

This chapter also reviews specific techniques for how the brain
can ease breathing discomfort and distress. These include mindful breathing and breathing retraining. Pursed-lips breathing is a
useful strategy that provides some relief as well as a sense of control when breathlessness develops. Lastly, yoga includes breathing as an integral part to control the mind and the body.

Anatomy of the Respiratory System

The respiratory system starts in your nose and mouth and ends
in the air sacs (alveoli; figure 1.1). Air enters the nose and mouth

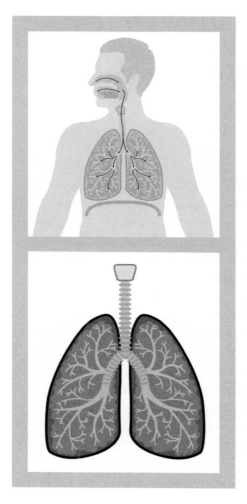

Figure 1.1 Pathway for inhaled air to enter the nose or mouth and pass through the windpipe (trachea) and the breathing tubes (airways) to reach the air sacs (alveoli). (Based on iStock.com images from elenabs and kowalska-art)

Figure 1.2 The vocal cords, windpipe (trachea), and breathing tubes (airways), which divide twenty-three times to end in air sacs (alveoli). (iStock.com/elenabs)

that join to form the throat (pharynx) and then passes through the voice box (larynx). The voice box consists of vocal cords that enable you to talk. Just below the voice box is the windpipe (trachea), which divides within the chest to form the right and left breathing tubes (airways). The entire system of breathing tubes is called the tracheobronchial tree because it looks like an upside-down tree.

Table 1.1 The upper respiratory system

STRUCTURE	MAJOR FUNCTIONS
Nose (hairs and turbinates*)	Warms, filters, and moistens inhaled air
	Detects odors
Mouth	Allows passage of air
Pharynx	Provides a resonating chamber for speech
	Epiglottis is a flap that prevents solids and liquids from entering the trachea and lungs
Larynx (vocal cords)	Makes sounds including speech

*Turbinates are long, narrowed, and curled bone shelves shaped like a seashell that protrudes into the breathing passage of the nose. Turbinates provide humidity for the lining of the nose that is needed for smell.

Table 1.2 The lower respiratory system

STRUCTURE	MAJOR FUNCTIONS
Trachea	Allows passage of air
Large and small airways	Allows passage of air
Alveoli	Gas exchange (oxygen enters the blood; carbon dioxide enters the air sacs or alveoli)

Overall, the breathing tubes (airways) divide twenty-three times as they go from large to small size tubes that end in air sacs (alveoli; figure 1.2).

The respiratory system is divided into upper and lower parts. The structures and major functions of the upper respiratory system are described in table 1.1.

The main structures and their functions of the lower respiratory tract are listed in table 1.2.

Normal Breathing

Most people do not think about their breathing as it is an unconscious action. Although you breathe ten to twelve times each minute, this happens without even a thought or concern. The size of each breath, called tidal volume, is about five hundred milliliters for an average size adult. This equals two cups of air (figure 1.3). Think about it: you breathe in and out two cups of air each breath that you take!

How does this happen? A group of nerve cells are located at the base of the brain that regularly sends electrical signals through nerves to the breathing muscles (figure 1.4).

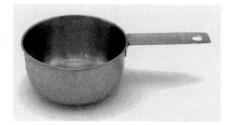

Figure 1.3 One-cup measuring container. The average breath is two cups of air. (iStock.com/sarahdoow)

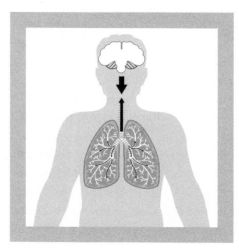

Figure 1.4 A group of nerves located in the lower part of the brain (brain stem) sends signals automatically to the breathing muscles that control how often we breathe and how deep. The upper part of the brain (cerebral cortex) has the ability to voluntarily control breathing. (Based on iStock.com images from elenabs and kowalska-art)

Figure 1.5 Shows the diaphragm, which is shaped like a dome and separates the chest and stomach (abdomen) cavities. (iStock.com/elenabs)

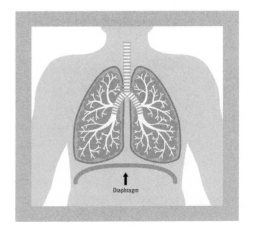

This is called the respiratory center and functions as a pacemaker for breathing. The right and left phrenic nerves (phrenic means "mind" in Latin) start in the neck (cervical nerves three through five) and pass down through the chest to each side of the diaphragm. The diaphragm is a muscle that is shaped like a dome. It is the main breathing muscle and separates the chest and the stomach (abdomen; figure 1.5).

The electrical signals that travel through the phrenic nerves tell the diaphragm when and how much to shorten (contract). When this happens, the dome-shaped diaphragm moves down toward the stomach cavity like a piston. Electrical signals also travel through other nerves to muscles located between ribs (called intercostal muscles). When the intercostal muscles shorten (contract), the ribs are lifted out to assist the diaphragm to breathe in air (figure 1.6).

If there is an even greater need to breathe in more air, electrical signals are also sent to neck muscles (called scalene and sternocleidomastoid muscles). When this happens the neck muscles shorten (contract) and lift the upper chest to breathe in more air (figure 1.7).

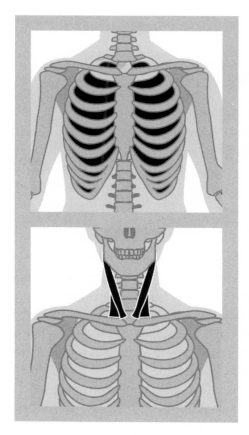

Figure 1.6 Each intercostal muscle connects an upper and lower rib on both sides of the chest. When these muscles shorten (contact), the ribs are lifted to help breathe in air. (iStock.com/elenabs)

Figure 1.7 Diagram of sternocleidomastoid muscles that connect the head and the upper chest. These muscles can assist breathing if necessary. (iStock.com/elenabs)

Voluntary Control of Breathing

The brain is able to override automatic breathing. This is called "voluntary control" as shown in figure 3.1. For example, you can decide to blow up a balloon or to hold your breath. This ability to voluntarily breathe more or breathe less when you want is unique to the respiratory system. No other part of the body can do this. Although the heart has a group of nerve cells that function as a pacemaker in order to control how many times the heart beats each minute, the brain cannot make the heart beat faster or slower!

Inspire

The word *inspire* means to inhale "good" air that contains 21 percent oxygen into our lungs. Air enters through the nose or mouth and travels through various passages (the upper and lower respiratory tracts) to reach the air sacs.

However, *inspire* also means to influence someone in a positive way. For example, a parent, teacher, or coach can inspire you to excel in learning a specific subject or skill. It is interesting that the word *inspire*, the act of breathing in, is linked to encouraging or producing a special feeling or thought in someone else.

Expire

The word *expire* means to exhale "bad" air (contains excess carbon dioxide) out of the lungs. At rest, exhaling air occurs because the elastic tissue in the lungs recoils inward just like a rubber band snaps back after it has been stretched. This recoil pressure forces air out through the breathing tubes and then out of the nose or mouth. With physical activities or exercise, certain stomach

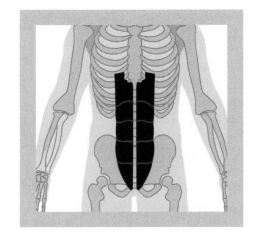

Figure 1.8 Diagram of the stomach muscles (called abdominal rectus). These muscles can assist in exhaling air with physical activities. (iStock.com/elenabs)

muscles (called abdominal rectus) and muscles that connect the ribs (called intercostal muscles) shorten to create positive pressure in the chest that helps to push air out of the lungs (figure 1.8).

Another meaning of *expire* is to give up life. In medical terms, it means that a person's breathing has stopped, and the person has died.

Mindful Breathing

Mindfulness is an ancient Buddhist practice that means paying attention to what is happening now. It is neither the past nor the future. "Stay in the moment" is a simple mantra that describes mindfulness. It is a practical way to notice not only breathing but also thoughts, sights, sounds, and smells—anything you might not normally consider.

The aim is to be mindful when performing everyday tasks such as eating, walking to the store, playing with grandchildren, waiting for a traffic light to turn green, or dealing with emotional challenges. Ideally, mindfulness is integrated into daily life in order to breathe easy and to support coping with shortness of breath and stress. The core principles of mindfulness can be applied as you cope with the challenges of living. These goals include the following:

Valuing self
Seeking and connecting with others
Seeing hardships as opportunities
Appreciating life
Being joyful
Adopting healthy behavior

With mindfulness, you can be in control of how you feel and how you approach each day.

Mindful breathing is an awareness of the physical act of breathing. Breathing in and out is something that you do, all of the time. By intentionally thinking about each breath, this can help you focus on the present. It is a simple way to allow you to be more aware of your body and its surroundings. Although the intent is to focus on each breath, it is likely that you will experience some wandering thoughts. This is fine and normal. It is important to notice the distractions and gently bring the focus back to breathing. Audio recordings are available that can provide guidance about mindful breathing. As your breathing becomes relaxed, then your muscles and entire body can also relax. The following are some suggestions for mindful breathing. Start this exercise for a few minutes and build up each day.

1 Sit quietly in a chair or lie down in bed before going to sleep.
2 Bring all of your attention to your breathing.
3 Notice that air enters your nose and travels to your lungs.
4 Consider whether the inward and outward breaths are warm or cool.
5 Notice that each time you breathe in, your stomach area moves out; and each time you breathe out, your stomach relaxes.
6 Remember that you don't need to do anything except be aware of breathing in and out.
7 It is okay if your thoughts wander. Just notice the thoughts and allow them to be, and bring your awareness back to your breathing.

If you or a family member has a medical condition, consider mindfulness as a deliberate approach to face the challenges of life, particularly breathing difficulty, no matter what else may be happening at the moment. With practice, mindful breathing can be used in times of breathing distress. If something happens that upsets you, consider mindful breathing as a strategy rather than smoking a cigarette or eating comfort food (figure 1.9).

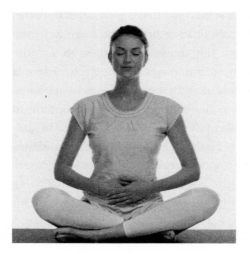

Figure 1.9 A person doing mindful breathing. (iStock.com/miljko)

Mindfulness can create an awareness of our body and release tension. A simple approach is to say to yourself, "Breathing in, I am aware of my body. Breathing out, I release stress and tension out of my body."

Breathing Retraining

The main focus of breathing retraining is to consciously breathe with the diaphragm rather than chest muscles. Other names for this are diaphragmatic breathing, abdominal breathing, and belly breathing. First, you should be in a comfortable position, either seated or lying down. Next, breathe in air through the nose by contracting the diaphragm muscle. Place the palm of one hand on the stomach area just below the ribs. With diaphragm breathing, you should feel the stomach pushing out as the diaphragm muscle moves down. As you exhale, you should feel the stomach area moving in as the diaphragm moves up. Many individuals use pursed-lips breathing when they perform diaphragmatic breathing (see below).

This approach is considered by some to be a healthy way to breathe and also provides a method to control and manage stress. Breathing retraining leads to an awareness of breathing as described for mindful breathing. When you first start to use breath retraining, you should practice it for five to ten minutes each day for a week. Once you are familiar with the technique, you should use it whenever you are aware of feeling stressed. Over time with regular practice, you should have a sense of a full, unrestricted breath that then becomes a normal feeling.

Pursed-Lips Breathing

Pursed-lips breathing is a simple three-step process that provides many benefits. Those with asthma or chronic obstructive pulmonary disease (COPD) either learn this technique on their own or are taught how to do pursed-lips breathing. The steps are illustrated in figure 1.10.

How does it work? The pressure created by puckering the lips helps to keep the breathing tubes from collapsing when you

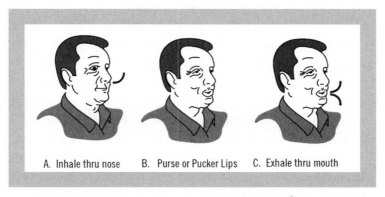

A. Inhale thru nose   B. Purse or Pucker Lips   C. Exhale thru mouth

Figure 1.10 Pursed-lips breathing is a three-step process: (1) Inhale slowly through your nose. (2) Pucker your lips together as to whistle. (3) Breathe out slowly through your mouth until all the air is out. (LeftRightCreative)

breathe out. The following benefits of pursed-lips breathing explain how it reduces the feeling of breathing difficulty:

Slows down breathing rate
Increases the amount of air exhaled in each breath that allows
    better emptying of the air (called lung deflation)
Increase oxygen saturation
Provides a sense of control of breathing

Mindful breathing can be combined with pursed-lips breathing to enhance the benefits and to ease breathing discomfort.

Yoga

Yoga is a form of physical movement and posture that includes meditation and spirituality. The word *yoga* means "to add," "to join," "to unite," or "to attach." Tibetan yoga emphasizes a continuous sequence of movement, whereas Indian yoga focuses on static positions.

Yoga is more than exercise as it is a technique for controlling the mind and body with breathing as an integral part. A popular form is called *hatha-yoga*, which focuses on physical and mental strength-building exercises, breathing, and meditation. Some mindfulness programs include yoga for relaxation and to reduce stress (figure 1.11).

Pay attention to your breathing right now. You will note that you breathe fast if you are upset or angry and breathe slow if you are calm and relaxed. This signifies that breathing is linked not only to the physical demands of the body but also to the mind. Stress and anxiety are major emotions that influence breathing. The practice of yoga encourages you to pay attention to breathing so you can bring your mind to a pleasant and peaceful state.

Pranayama is a traditional yoga practice of controlling the breath. Although there are many forms of breathing strategies

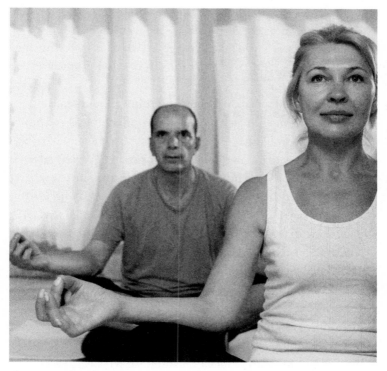

Figure 1.11 Couple in yoga pose. (iStock.com/JackF)

used in yoga, in general the focus is on slowing and extending the breath, particularly during meditation. Yoga emphasizes that when you breathe in, you bring in energy (you are inhaling oxygen) to your body, and when you breathe out, you allow stress to leave your body (you are exhaling carbon dioxide).

There is evidence that yoga is beneficial for those with heart disease, stroke, and COPD. In a review article of ten studies (a total of 431 individuals with average age being fifty-six), those who performed yoga increased their exercise capacity as well as their quality of life. You may wish to give yoga a try by itself or in addition to a standard rehabilitation program.

Key Points

> With each breath, you take in oxygen—which is necessary for life—and you get rid of carbon dioxide, a waste product of the body.
> Breathing is unconscious. You don't think about breathing unless someone brings it to your attention or unless you have a breathing problem.
> *Inspire* means to inhale "good" air (21 percent oxygen) into the lungs and also to influence someone in a positive way. It is interesting that the act of life—breathing—is linked to encouraging or producing a special feeling in someone else.
> *Expire* means to breathe "bad" air out of the lungs. This eliminates excess carbon dioxide. *Expire* also means to come to an end, such as an expiration date or death.
> Mindful breathing allows you be more aware of the present. "Stay in the moment" captures the principle of mindfulness.
> Breathing retraining involves conscious use of the diaphragm when breathing in.
> Pursed-lips breathing is a simple three-step process that reduces the feeling of breathing difficulty. It can be used along with mindful breathing and breathing retraining.
> Yoga is a technique for connecting the mind and the body using breathing as an integral part.

References

Benzo, Roberto P. "Mindfulness and Motivational Interviewing: Two Candidate Methods for Promoting Self-Management." *Chronic Respiratory Disease* 10 (2013): 175–82.

CioffrediPT. "Learn the Diaphragmatic Breathing Technique." YouTube, August 22, 2012. https://www.youtube.com/.

Desveaux, Laura, Annemarie Lee, Roger Goldstein, and Dina Brooks. "Yoga in the Management of Chronic Disease: A Systematic Review and Meta-analysis." *Medical Care* 53 (July 2015): 653–61.

Kabat-Zinn, Jon. *Wherever You Go, There You Are: Mindfulness Meditation in Everyday Life.* New York: Hyperion, 1994.

Payne, Rosemary. *Relaxation Techniques: A Practical Guide for the Health Care Professional.* 3rd ed. Edinburgh: Elsevier Churchill Livingstone, 2005.

(2)

Second Wind

A bull . . . if allowed to get its "second wind" . . .
will go on almost forever.
Anonymous, 1893

George is sixty-three years old and was diagnosed with chronic obstructive pulmonary disease (COPD) about four years ago. He retired recently as a dispatcher for a car service. His COPD medications include an inhaled long-acting bronchodilator as well as albuterol when needed.

Over the past year, he noticed that his breathing was more difficult when doing yard work and walking his dog, particularly up inclines, or any activity that required prolonged exertion. At a recent medical appointment, George told the physician's assistant (PA) that his shortness of breath was getting worse. Breathing tests and a chest x-ray showed that his COPD was stable, and the PA recommended that George start a pulmonary rehabilitation program at the local hospital.

George agreed and discussed his goals with the coordinator. The coordinator suggested that George monitor his exercise intensity (how hard to push) by using either a target level of breathlessness on a zero-to-ten scale or by using a target heart rate. He attended three sessions each week that included walking on the treadmill, pedaling on a stationary cycle, and using a rowing machine. George worked hard and gradually increased the workloads and total exercise times. After a few weeks, George noted that his breathing was getting easier doing the exercises and daily activities. In the fifth week of rehabilitation, George wanted to see if he could walk on the treadmill for thirty minutes without stopping (his previous best was eighteen minutes). After about ten to twelve minutes on the treadmill, George sensed that his breathing was getting easy and he felt strong. After completing the thirty-minute session, he immediately shared this feeling with the program co-ordinator who suggested that George has experienced "second wind." In thinking about this, George remembered the same feeling decades ago when he ran cross-country in high school.

What Is Second Wind?

"Second wind" is a person's ability to breathe freely during exercise, after having been out of breath. It is commonly associated with renewed energy or strength. One person described it as follows: "To me, it just feels like I have something left in the tank. It's a confidence that, between energy stores and breathing, I feel like I can finish."

Your first experience of "second wind" may have occurred when you were younger while playing sports. If you have a chronic lung condition, such as asthma or COPD, it is possible that you may have noticed a "second wind" during a pulmonary rehabilitation session as George did. Although "second wind" may be hard to explain to others, most everyone agrees that experiencing a "second wind" is a pleasant feeling.

If you have not experienced "second wind," consider that the start of exercise can be associated with feeling sluggish and slow to move; it may even be hard to breathe. These initial feelings may be unpleasant, perhaps even making you think about stopping or "giving up." However, if you are able to continue, the motions of your arms, legs, and entire body may become more fluid and your energy level may rise. It is possible, even likely, that breathing becomes easier.

Another definition refers to a second burst of strength or energy after you feel tired and unsure whether you are able to continue.

For example, you might be tired and short of breath from doing housework, doing yard work, or taking a hike. This sense of fatigue and breathing difficulty may also occur while walking on the treadmill or pedaling a stationary cycle at a pulmonary rehabilitation session. If you decide to keep going, hopefully you will have more energy and confidence in completing the task.

Second Wind and Running

Many articles about "second wind" relate to running. Some runners describe feeling stronger and breathing easier about ten to fifteen minutes into a run. One runner explained the feeling as follows: "Your body is telling your mind, I can do this." Unfortunately, runners report that they never know when to expect this experience, and it doesn't happen on every run. In fact, it may be hard to predict.

The late Dr. George Sheehan, a cardiologist who wrote about the joy and benefits of running in the 1970s and 1980s, advised runners "to wait for your second wind." He described it as follows: "It takes 6 to 10 minutes and one degree in body temperature to shunt the blood to the working muscles. When that happens, you will experience a light warm sweat and know what the 'second wind' means."

Author and runner Hal Higdon commented that in the middle of a run he might feel exhilaration that he also described as "second wind" or "runner's high." He commented that the feeling was like "leaving the cares of the world behind you."

What Causes Second Wind?

Actually, no one knows for sure what causes second wind. Scientific studies do not provide a definite answer. Four different possibilities have been proposed:

1 Use of fat as a fuel for energy (fat burn)
2 Steady state
3 Release of endorphins
4 Psychological

To perform any activity, our muscles require oxygen and energy (fuel for the body). The three sources of energy are carbohydrates, fats, and protein. The fat-burn theory refers to switching, or changing, from carbohydrate (glycogen) as a fuel for the exercising muscles to the use of fat. This switching process has been observed in a rare muscle condition (called McArdle's disease), and a similar phenomenon may occur in individuals to explain "second wind."

Another possible reason is that the body achieves a metabolic balance (steady state) or equilibrium during exertion. As the muscles warm up and the body temperature increases slightly, our breathing is able to supply enough oxygen to meet the demands of the muscles. At this point in exercise, our muscles become more efficient, breathing evens out, and fatigue may disappear. Physiologists call this "steady state."

A third explanation for "second wind" is the release of chemicals called endorphins into the brain. Endorphins are naturally occurring narcotics that act in the brain to make us "feel good" by taking away pain and breathing difficulty. Studies show that endorphins are released during exercise in healthy individuals and also in those with COPD. These narcotic-like substances clearly make it easier to breathe and may contribute to "second wind." Endocannabinoids are another type of chemical that is elevated with exercise. These substances are similar to marijuana and can affect mood and the sensation of pain. There is wide variation in how a person responds to endorphins and endocannabinoids. So, it is difficult to predict who will experience "second wind," when it will happen, and how it will feel.

A final consideration is that "second wind" is entirely psycho-logical. It may be a by-product of confidence and pride as you achieve more than is expected. This may also occur if you receive encouragement from a coach, a physical therapist, or a pulmo-nary rehabilitation coordinator while you are exercising.

From a practical perspective, it really does not matter what causes "second wind." More importantly, "second wind" is a posi-tive breathing experience when it happens, and you should enjoy it.

Second Wind and Chronic Lung Disease

If you have a chronic lung condition, think about whether you have ever experienced "second wind." Scientists suggest that "second wind" occurs when a physical activity lasts for at least ten minutes. Some individuals with asthma or COPD have told me that they have experienced a "second wind" while doing any sus-tained activity such as housework, yard work, walking, and hiking. Certainly, you won't experience second wind if you stop doing the activity when your breathing starts to be uncomfortable.

The ten-minute requirement is a reason that those participat-ing in pulmonary rehabilitation have the best chance of experi-encing a "second wind." The sessions are supervised by a trained professional who monitors your body's responses (heart rate, breathing, and oxygen level) and also provides encouragement to do more than you did last session or last week. The entire expe-rience provides an environment for safely "pushing yourself" to exercise beyond the ten minutes in order to hopefully experience a "second wind."

A Second-Wind Approach to Life

A Google search reveals at least two books that include "second wind" in the title. Both books describe a journey about a "fresh start" or achieving a more meaningful life. In 2008, Jan Tilley wrote *Getting Your Second Wind* about finding a personal path to wellness and tapping into motivation. She proposed deliberately making healthy choices in diet, exercise, and mental outlook to enjoy "a powerful transformation" in order to find personal fulfillment. In 2014, Dr. Bill Thomas wrote about *Navigating the Passage to a Slower, Deeper, and More Connected Life*, as a way to achieve a *Second Wind*, the title of his book. Thomas describes the need to "fix" the feeling that life is out of balance and no longer fulfilling. His emphasis is on needing to "de-stress and rethink" our lives, particularly for those over fifty years of age.

These two books illustrate that "second wind" can have a more general meaning of slowing down and focusing on what is meaningful in your life. Thomas writes that reexamination is important "when the need to perform, to hurry, and to acquire is no longer compelling."

Key Points

> "Second wind" refers to the return of relatively easier breathing after initial fatigue or exhaustion during exertion.
> The experience of a "second wind" generally takes at least ten minutes of continuous exercise before it occurs.
> "Second wind" can also mean a renewed energy past the point of fatigue or tiredness. It means to regain one's strength.
> In a book written by Dr. Bill Thomas, "second wind" refers to reconnecting to what is meaningful in your life and finding the right balance on a daily basis.

References

Higdon, Hal. *Hal Higdon's Smart Running*. Emmaus, PA: Rodale, 1998.
Sheehan, George. "Important Running Tips for Every Runner to Know."

DrGeorgeSheehan, accessed September 20, 2016. http://www
.georgesheehan.com/.

Thomas, Bill. *Second Wind: Navigating the Passage to a Slower, Deeper, and More Connected Life*. New York: Simon & Schuster, 2014.

Tilley, Jan. *Getting Your Second Wind*. Tucson: Wheatmark, 2008.

(3)

Why Am I Short of Breath?

If you want to conquer the anxiety of life,

live in the moment, live in the breath.

Amit Ray, author of books on meditation (1960–)

Breathing difficulty, commonly called shortness of breath, is a common complaint, especially if you have a heart or lung condition. Many individuals find that it is hard to describe the actual feeling of difficult breathing. Also, you may assume that any shortness of breath is due to getting older, or being out of shape. Or, you may be afraid to find out that you have a medical problem that could seriously affect your health.

Individuals frequently delay seeking medical attention until their trouble breathing interferes with doing physical tasks, such as housework, yard work, or shopping. Another factor is how much effort you are willing to exert in order to complete the activity. For example, you may decide that it is too challenging or too exhausting to walk up a flight of stairs even though you know you could do so if necessary. Or, you may decide to play nine holes of golf instead of eighteen holes in order to conserve energy and to reduce the demands on breathing.

If you experience shortness of breath or breathing difficulty with any activities, make sure to tell your health-care provider. Be sure to describe when the breathing problem started, what activities bring on the difficulty, and what, if anything, you do to make it better. Also, consider this question: have you have stopped doing anything because it is too hard to breathe?

This chapter describes why you might experience shortness of breath (the medical word is *dyspnea*). This information provides a simple explanation of how a heart or lung condition can cause the feeling that it is hard or difficult to breathe. In medical terms, this is called the *neurobiology of dyspnea*, or how the brain (neuro-) and respiratory system (-biology) interact to cause breathing difficulty. The five common conditions that cause shortness of breath are reviewed using a simple question-and-answer format:

1 What is the condition?
2 What are the major causes of the condition?
3 How does each condition cause shortness of breath?
4 How is each condition diagnosed?

In each of these medical problems, breathing difficulty typically develops slowly over months or even years. It is important to understand how each condition actually causes shortness of breath as many individuals assume that a breathing problem is due to a low oxygen level. Although a low oxygen level can certainly cause breathing difficulty, it is not that simple.

Why Does Shortness of Breath Occur?

To answer this question, it is important to understand how the brain and the respiratory system communicate. This is illustrated in figure 3.1. There are numerous sensors called receptors that send electrical signals through nerves (primarily the vagal nerve) to the brain. Theses receptors are located in the neck, the lungs, and the muscles of the chest that provide information about many things including the oxygen level in the blood and how the lungs are working. Normally, there is a "match" or agreement between the signals going to the brain from the respiratory system and those going from the brain down to the breathing muscles. If there is a good match, you are not aware of your breathing. The system is working fine, and breathing is unconscious.

However, if there is a "mismatch" between signals (respiratory

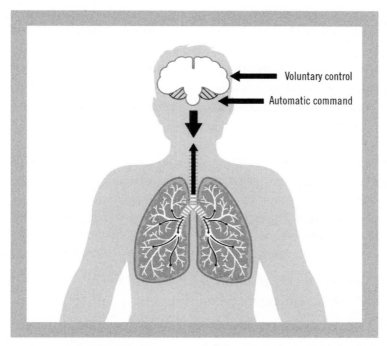

Figure 3.1 Upward arrows show signals being sent from the respiratory system up to the brain. These electrical signals come from sensors in parts of the lung and are sent through nerves to reach the brain. Downward arrow represents signals sent from the brain to the breathing muscles to breathe more. The upper part of the brain (cerebral cortex) enables a person to hold the breath (at least for a while) or to breathe faster and deeper. This is called voluntary control. (Based on iStock.com images from elenabs and kowalska-art)

system → brain → respiratory system), then you become aware of a feeling that it is hard or difficult to breathe. For example, if you develop pneumonia, sensors in the lungs send signals to the brain; in response, the brain sends strong signals to the respiratory system to breathe more to try to compensate. This creates a mismatch or disagreement between the signals from the brain and the respiratory system. In addition, pneumonia can reduce the level of oxygen in the blood. A sensor in each side of the neck (called the carotid body) informs the brain to breathe faster and deeper in an effort to take in more oxygen and correct the problem. With pneumonia, there are two different pathways that can cause you to feel short of breath.

Research studies have shown that you may experience breathing difficulty in different ways. For example, you may feel the *intensity* of shortness of breath, or how bad the breathing seems. Another experience is how *unpleasant* your breathing seems. There are different sensors and nerve pathways that provide unique information from the respiratory system to different parts of the brain for the experiences of intensity and unpleasantness of breathlessness.

What Will My Health-Care Provider Do to Find the Cause of My Shortness of Breath?

Certainly, there are many illnesses that can cause breathing difficulty. However, heart and lung diseases are the most common reasons. Usually, your health-care provider will be able to find the cause or reason for your shortness of breath using a standard approach: asking many questions (medical history), performing a physical examination, and ordering tests.

Usually the nurse or medical assistant will measure how much oxygen is in your blood by placing a medical device on your finger. The device is called an oximeter and is shown in figure 3.2. It

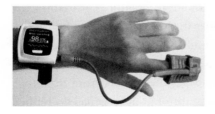

Figure 3.2 Photo of device called pulse oximeter placed on a finger to measure oxygen saturation in the blood. The device works by sensing each pulse from the heart. (Wikimedia Commons)

is simple and noninvasive. The device passes two waves of light through the finger that measure the percentage of hemoglobin, the protein in the red blood cell that carries oxygen. The value is called oxygen saturation (abbreviated SpO2), and a normal value is 95 percent or higher. A SpO2 below 95 percent suggests a problem between oxygen reaching the air sacs (called alveoli) in the lung and the flow of blood passing next to the air sacs (called pulmonary capillaries). A value of 88 percent or below means that you should use oxygen.

It is important to know that there are some limitations if you use an oximeter at home and check your own saturation level. The device is not accurate if there is poor blood flow to the finger. This can happen if you finger or hand is cold, or if you are moving a lot, like shivering. There should be a steady pulse for the device to be accurate. For example, if you have an irregular heart rhythm, such as atrial fibrillation, the recorded value may be inconsistent.

What Conditions Cause Shortness of Breath?

The five common conditions that can cause shortness of breath are presented in alphabetical order. Knowing about these causes can help you understand the reasons for your breathing difficulty.

ANEMIA

What Is Anemia? Anemia means a low number of red blood cells. Red blood cells are made in the bone marrow and then released into the blood.

What Are the Major Causes of Anemia? Red blood cells live for 120 days. Your bone marrow must continually make new red blood cells to replace the old ones that die. One major reason for anemia is the failure of the bone marrow to produce enough red blood cells. This could be due to low intake of certain vitamins and iron or a chronic medical condition such as kidney failure in which the bone marrow does not work normally. Also, certain medications can depress the function of the bone marrow.

Another common cause for anemia is loss of blood from the body. This can happen if you have menstrual periods, if you had major injury or trauma, if you had surgery, or if you bleed from your stomach (ulcer or cancer) or from your intestines (polyps or cancer).

How Does Anemia Cause Shortness of Breath? Red blood cells carry oxygen to all parts of the body. With fewer red blood cells (anemia), there is less oxygen available, and cells may not work normally. This is particularly a problem when you do physical tasks or exercise because active muscles require more oxygen than muscles at rest.

The body attempts to compensate for the low amount of oxygen in the blood by two major responses: You breathe more in an attempt to inhale more oxygen into the body. And your heart beats faster in an attempt to deliver more oxygen to the muscles. As a result of the increased breathing, you likely feel short of breath.

How Is Anemia Diagnosed? A blood test called a complete blood count (CBC) is required to identify whether you have anemia. The specific cause of anemia requires additional testing of the blood. Your health-care provider may refer you to a specialist in blood diseases—called a hematologist. Sometimes, a sample of the bone marrow is obtained to learn more about possible causes of anemia.

ANXIETY

What Is Anxiety? Anxiety is a general feeling of worry, apprehension, irritability, and restlessness. You may feel afraid and be overly concerned about health, money, family relations, work, school, or being in various social situations. It is common that you may have trouble both identifying the specific fear and controlling these feelings. The fear is usually magnified compared with the reality of what is happening. Anxiety is considered a problem when symptoms interfere with a person's ability to function and to sleep.

In addition to these feelings, physical signs of anxiety are a result of the body's *fight or flight* response. Common symptoms include the heart pounding, sweating, frequent urination or diarrhea, shortness of breath, fatigue, and trouble sleeping. Sometimes, those who suffer from anxiety may mistake their symptoms for a medical illness.

What Are the Major Causes of Anxiety? Anxiety is commonly triggered by stress. Usually anxiety is a response to outside forces, including death of a loved one, difficulties in a personal relationship, stress at work or school, and concerns about money. It is possible to become anxious with "negative self-talk." This means telling yourself that the worst is going to happen. You may experience a general state of worry or fear before doing something challenging such as taking a test, going for a job interview, attending a reception, or having an appointment with a health-care professional. In addition, just feeling short of breath from any condition can be scary and contribute to feeling anxious.

How Does Anxiety Cause Shortness of Breath? Anxiety is a feeling of discomfort. If you have a high level of anxiety, you may feel it is hard to breathe at rest or when talking. Typically, anxiety causes you to breathe faster and often deeper. This is called hyperventilation, and others may notice that you are breathing this way. At times, anxiety may become so severe to cause panic and a feeling that you are losing control.

How Is Anxiety Diagnosed? The diagnosis depends on you reporting exactly how you feel. Common symptoms are feeling nervous, uncomfortable, and jittery. You may also feel restless and perspire easily. Those who experience high anxiety often feel that their breathing is frightening or awful. Another common complaint is that it is "hard to get enough air in." If you experience any of these feelings about breathing, you should tell your health-care professional.

A family member or friend may observe that you appear uncomfortable or may be aware that you worry about everything. Your health-care provider may recommend therapy and also refer you to a specialist—either a psychologist or psychiatrist. These professionals can use specific questionnaires to help diagnose anxiety.

DECONDITIONING

What Is Deconditioning? Deconditioning is a low level of fitness, or in simple terms, being out of shape. When this happens, your heart and lungs become less efficient, especially with physical activities.

What Are the Major Causes of Deconditioning? Deconditioning is a direct result of reduced physical activities over a period of time. There are many reasons someone gets out of shape:

Too busy with work or family
Feeling tired or lazy so that you don't want to do anything
Being depressed
An illness (such as the flu or arthritis) or a chest infection
   (bronchitis or pneumonia)
An injury (e.g., a broken bone or a sprained ankle)
An operation (e.g., a knee or hip replacement)

If you have shortness of breath for any reason, it is quite common to reduce physical activities to avoid this unpleasant experience. This inactivity creates a downward spiral that contributes to more shortness of breath as illustrated in figure 3.3. Deconditioning can happen if you are otherwise healthy or may develop if you have a heart or lung disease and then make your shortness of breath even worse.

How Does Deconditioning Cause Shortness of Breath? If you become deconditioned, your heart and lungs must work harder to

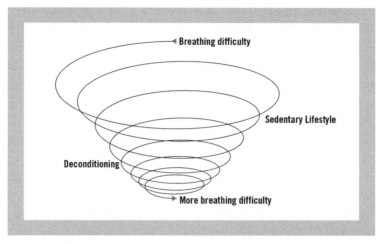

Figure 3.3 Downward spiral showing that inactivity leads to deconditioning and then shortness of breath. This downward spiral continues if you further reduce physical activities. (LeftRightCreative)

deliver oxygen to all parts of the body. This means that even at rest your heart beats faster and you must breathe more. The demands on your heart and lungs are even greater with physical activities when your muscles demand more oxygen. To take in more oxygen, you breathe in deeper and more frequently. This leads to the typical experience of feeling "out of breath."

How Is Deconditioning Diagnosed? You can suspect deconditioning as a cause for your breathing difficulty by simply considering a few questions about your current and previous activities. Do you go for walks? Do you perform housework or yard work? Do you walk up a flight of stairs or take an elevator instead? Do you use a gym or fitness center? Have you had a recent injury or illness? Did you have an operation in the past few months? Also, have you gained weight? As you become deconditioned, the body's metabolism slows down and you burn fewer calories as you are less active.

Activity monitors (wrist bands and smartphones) can estimate how many steps you take or how many calories you use each day. This information can provide a clue about your daily activities. A more specific way to diagnose deconditioning is an exercise test. This involves exercise on a treadmill or stationary cycle while your heart and breathing are monitored. Your fitness can be measured by the amount of work you perform during exercise and by measuring how much oxygen your body uses during the test. The exercise test is also a way to determine whether you have any evidence of heart or lung disease.

HEART DISEASE

What Is Heart Disease? Heart disease is a general term for a condition that affects the normal function of the heart.

What Are the Major Causes of Heart Disease? The three major causes of heart disease are as follows:

The blood vessels in the heart become narrow and blocked
    (called coronary artery disease).
One of the four heart valves either becomes too tight and limits
    the flow of blood (called stenosis) or does not close completely
    and allows blood to flow backward (called regurgitation).
    These situations are called valvular heart disease.
The heart muscle becomes weak and is unable to normally pump
    blood to parts of the body (called myocardial disease).

Both narrowing and blockage of the blood vessels of the heart and weak heart muscles affect the pumping action of the heart. Heart-valve problems put an extra strain on the heart.

There are several risk factors that cause narrowing to occur in the blood vessels of the heart. These include

high levels of cholesterol and other fats in the blood,
smoking,
high blood pressure,

diabetes mellitus, and
inflammation in the blood vessels of the heart.

Plaque can develop inside the blood vessels of the heart due to one or more of the risk factors (figure 3.4). Plaque buildup may start as early as childhood. Over time, the plaque may harden or break open (rupture). If it ruptures, blood cells called platelets stick to the site of rupture forming a clot that can block the blood flow to the heart muscle (figure 3.5).

Any of the four valves of the heart may be defective at birth, can be damaged if bacteria in the blood attaches to one of the valves (called endocarditis), or may "wear out" with aging. More than one in ten people over seventy-five years of age have a heart valve problem.

Diseases of the heart muscles (called cardiomyopathy) limit the ability of these muscles to pump blood. This typically leads to a buildup of fluid in the lungs called congestive heart failure, which causes shortness of breath. This condition increases the risk of irregular heart rhythms and sudden death. Possible diseases of the heart muscles include a genetic disorder; an infection such as hepatitis C; toxic effects of alcohol abuse, diabetes, or an overactive thyroid (called hyperthyroidism); and obesity.

How Does Heart Disease Cause Shortness of Breath? One of the chambers on the left side of the heart (called the left ventricle) pumps blood to all parts of the body including the brain, internal organs, and muscles. If the pumping action does not work as it should, fluid may back up into the lungs. This is just like a plugged drainage pipe causing backup of fluids into the sink. This backup causes fluid to accumulate in the air sacs of the lungs and activates sensors that send signals to the brain that there is a problem. This process of fluid in the lungs is called congestive heart failure.

How Is Heart Disease Diagnosed? Your health-care provider may detect a problem by listening to your heart using a stethoscope.

Figure 3.4 Views inside a blood vessel. The top view shows normal blood flow. The bottom view shows narrowing of the blood vessel due to plaque buildup. The plaque buildup reduces blood flow. (iStock.com/stock_shoppe)

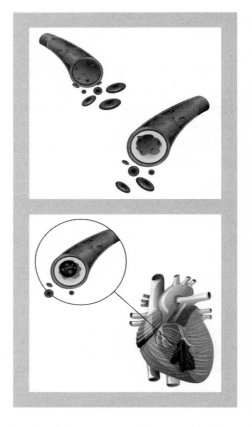

Figure 3.5 View of the heart and a blood vessel of the heart. The inside of the blood vessel shows plaque buildup. With rupture of the plaque, platelets stick to the rupture area in an attempt to repair the injury. However, a blood clot can form and block blood flow to the heart muscle. Reduced blood flow can cause chest pain (called angina) and a heart attack (called myocardial infarction). Poor blood flow to the heart muscles can also interfere with the pumping action of the heart, leading to a backup of fluid into the lungs that causes shortness of breath. (Based on iStock.com images from rabbit team and stock_shoppe)

An electrocardiogram is frequently obtained to assess your heart rhythm (is the heart beating regularly or irregularly?) and to look for signs of abnormal function. Usually, an echocardiogram is ordered; this is a noninvasive test using sound waves (called ultrasound) to visualize the heart valves and the function of the heart muscles.

Your health-care provider may refer you to a specialist in heart diseases—called a cardiologist. The cardiologist may decide to perform a catheterization of the blood vessels to determine whether you have a blockage in one or more of the blood vessels in the heart or to visualize the heart valves. For this test, a plastic flexible tube is inserted in the groin or arm vein and then passed into the heart; dye is injected through the tube in order to look for blockage in the blood vessels of the heart (called coronary arteries).

LUNG DISEASE

What Is Lung Disease? Lung disease is a general term for a condition that affects the normal function of the respiratory system.

What Are the Major Causes of Lung Disease? Different conditions or diseases can affect any part of the respiratory system. The major diseases of the respiratory system are listed in table 3.1.

The various conditions listed in this table show that there are many diseases that involve or affect the respiratory system. Your health-care provider needs to consider all of these possible causes for shortness of breath.

How Does Lung Disease Cause Shortness of Breath? Any lung disease can activate sensors that send signals to alert the brain of a problem (as discussed earlier in the chapter). For example, a low oxygen level in the blood activates sensors in the neck (a collection of nerve cells called the carotid body). Figure 3.6 shows the location of the carotid body. When the carotid body is activated by a low oxygen level in the blood, it sends electrical signals to the brain. Then, the brain sends signals down to the respiratory system to "breathe more" in an attempt to increase the oxygen level.

In those with asthma, sensors in the breathing tubes (airways) can be stimulated to cause breathing difficulty and chest tightness (figure 3.7). In those with chronic obstructive pulminary disease (COPD), sensors in the breathing muscles can be activated as a direct result of not being able to exhale the normal amount of

Table 3.1 Major diseases that involve or affect
the respiratory system

LOCATION	DISEASE
Upper airway	Vocal cord dysfunction
	Stenosis (narrowing) of the trachea
	Goiter (enlarged thyroid gland)
Airways (breathing tubes)	Asthma
	Chronic obstructive pulmonary disease (COPD)
Lungs	Lung cancer
	Bronchiectasis (dilated breathing tubes) usually with a chronic lung infection
	Interstitial lung disease (inflammation or fibrosis [scarring] in the lungs)
	Lung cancer
Chest wall	Kyphoscoliosis (curvature of the spine)
	Obesity
	Pleural effusion (fluid in the lining around the lung)
Respiratory muscles	Paralysis of diaphragm
	Neuromuscular disease (e.g., muscular dystrophy)
	Myopathy (muscle weakness)
Blood vessels	Pulmonary hypertension (high blood pressure in the blood vessels of the lungs)
	Pulmonary embolism (blood clots to the lungs)

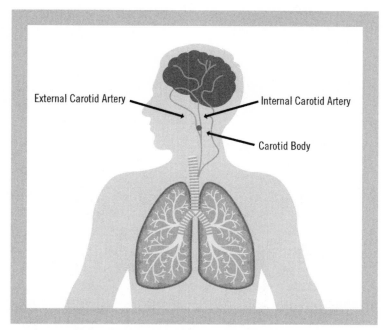

Figure 3.6 The carotid artery is located in the neck and provides blood from the aorta to the brain. It divides into internal and external branches. The carotid body (a group of nerve cells) is located where the internal and external branches start.

air out the lungs. This trapped air (called hyperinflation) pushes the diaphragm muscle down, making it less efficient when taking a breath in (figure 3.8).

How Is Lung Disease Diagnosed? Most likely, your health-care provider will ask you what activities bring on breathing difficulty and what you do to make it better. Also, consider if you have stopped doing some activities because it is too hard to breathe. You will likely be asked if you have other chest symptoms such as a dry cough, a cough that raises mucus, wheezing, chest tightness, or breathing difficulty when you sleep. As examples, a feeling that "my chest feels tight" is suggestive of asthma; or a feeling that "my

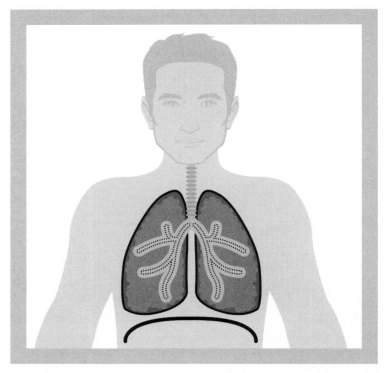

Figure 3.7 Sensors line the inside of the breathing tubes. When these breathing tubes constrict, or tighten, as shown by the dashed lines, sensors are activated. Electrical signals are sent to the brain, which has the experience of chest tightness. This process is most common in those with asthma. (Based on iStock.com images from elenabs and kowalska-art)

breathing is shallow" raises the possibility of interstitial lung disease. As inhaling dusts, fibers, fumes, or other airborne irritants can cause lung disease, you will likely be asked about your work history and hobbies.

Breathing tests (called pulmonary function tests [PFTS]) and a chest x-ray are the usual starting points for figuring out a specific respiratory diagnosis. If the breathing tests are normal, two additional tests may be ordered by your health-care provider: a metha-

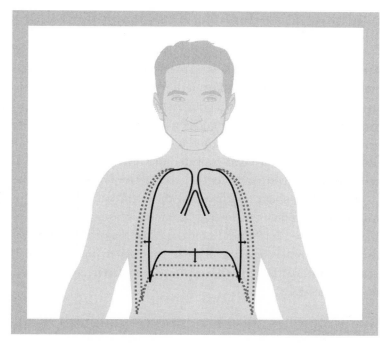

Figure 3.8 As a result of narrowing, or obstruction, of the breathing tubes, the normal amount of air cannot be exhaled out of the lungs. Air is then trapped in the lungs, which push the diaphragm muscle down. This is called hyperinflation as noted by arrows facing out and down. This process can activate sensors in the diaphragm and other chest muscles to cause shortness of breath. (Based on iStock.com images from elenabs and kowalska-art)

choline challenge test—a specific breathing test for asthma; and a cardiopulmonary exercise test to measure the responses of the heart and lungs to the demands of exercise.

Sometimes a CT (computerized tomography) scan of the chest is ordered, especially if lung cancer, interstitial lung disease, or blood clots to the lungs are considered. Various blood tests are usually ordered to evaluate for specific types of interstitial lung disease and pulmonary hypertension.

Summary

This chapter describes the five most common chronic (present for at least a few months) causes for shortness of breath. It is important to realize that this information does not cover all possible causes. Rather, this chapter highlights five conditions that you and your health-care provider should consider when starting to figure out why you are short of breath. If initial testing does not provide an answer, your health-care provider may refer you to a lung (pulmonologist) or heart (cardiologist) specialist for further evaluation.

Information about treatment for these different causes is not provided in this chapter. Such information is beyond the scope of the book. However, therapies for the three major chronic respiratory conditions—asthma, chronic obstructive pulmonary disease, and interstitial lung disease—are included in chapters 4, 5, and 7 respectively.

Key Points

> Shortness of breath is due to a "mismatch" between signals sent from sensors in the respiratory system to the brain and the signals sent from the brain to the breathing muscles to breathe deeper and faster.
> If you experience breathing difficulty, tell your health-care provider. It is important to find out the cause of your problem as treatment will likely help.
> The major conditions that cause chronic shortness of breath are anemia, anxiety, deconditioning, heart diseases, and lung disease.
> Your health-care provider should be able to find the cause of your breathing difficulty by asking appropriate questions, by doing a physical examination, and by ordering various tests.
> By understanding the information in this chapter, you can

assist your health-care provider in answering the question "Why am I short of breath?"

References

Chang, Andrew S., Jeffrey Munson, Alex H. Gifford, and Donald A. Mahler. "Prospective Use of Descriptors of Dyspnea to Diagnose Common Respiratory Diseases." *Chest* 148 (2015): 895–902.

Gifford, Alex H., and Donald A. Mahler. "Chronic Dyspnea." In *Dyspnea: Mechanisms, Measurement, and Management*, edited by Donald A. Mahler and Denis E. O'Donnell, 145–63. 3rd ed. Boca Raton, FL: CRC Press, 2014.

Mahler, Donald A., and Denis E. O'Donnell. "Recent Advances in Dyspnea." *Chest* 147 (2015): 232–39.

(4)

Asthma

Asthma doesn't seem to bother me any more unless
I'm around cigars or dogs. The thing that would bother
me most would be a dog smoking a cigar.
Steve Allen, comedian (1921–2000)

Asthma is a disease of the breathing tubes (airways) that affects
more than twenty-five million Americans. About six million of
these are children. The key characteristics of asthma are redness
and swelling of the breathing tubes (inflammation); narrowing of
the breathing tubes (airway obstruction); and increased tendency
for breathing tubes to narrow or constrict (bronchoconstriction).
Figure 4.1 shows the important role of inflammation that leads to
other features of asthma.

Preventing and treating inflammation is the key target to obtain good asthma control. However, a successful response to therapy may take weeks to achieve and may be incomplete. For some
individuals, chronic inflammation is associated with permanent
damage to the breathing tubes. This is called "airway remodeling"
and can limit the response to asthma therapies.

Why Does Someone Develop Asthma?

There is no simple answer to this question. It is generally believed that it occurs when someone who has an increased risk
for having asthma (called genetic susceptibility) is exposed to a
"trigger" or "insult" at a crucial time. For example, a child whose
mother or father has asthma may develop the problem when a
"chest cold" occurs or when exposed to an allergen in the environ-

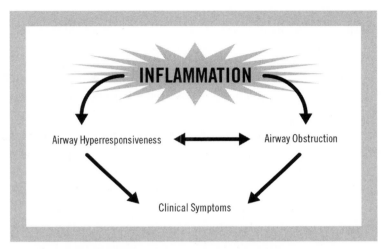

Figure 4.1 Inflammation of the breathing tubes causes airway obstruction (narrowing) and airway hyperresponsiveness (tendency for bronchoconstriction). These lead to shortness of breath, wheezing, cough, and chest tightness—the symptoms of asthma. (LeftRightCreative)

ment, such as house dust mites or cat dander. It is interesting that in early life, asthma is more common in boys, while at puberty, asthma predominates in females. This observation suggests that sex hormones such as estrogen may contribute to the onset and persistence of the disease.

Inflammation

Inflammation plays a key role in asthma. There are many types of inflammatory cells in the breathing tubes that contribute to differences in severity and response to therapy. The major types of inflammatory cells in asthma are as follows:

Lymphocytes: may determine scarring of the breathing tubes (airway remodeling);
Mast cells: release mediators that cause bronchoconstriction;

Eosinophils: correlate with asthma severity; and

Neutrophils: increased in those with severe asthma and in those who smoke.

Why is this important? First, the type of inflammatory cell may be quite different among those who have asthma. As examples, the eosinophil (figure 4.2) tends to be the major inflammatory cell in those who have allergies associated with their asthma, whereas the neutrophil dominates in those with more severe asthma who are past or active smokers. At the present time, it is only possible to identify those individuals with high numbers of eosinophils by simple tests—either blood tests or tests analyzing exhaled air. A biopsy sample of the breathing tubes is required to identify the other types of inflammatory cells, but this is only done in research studies. Second, different medications target different inflammatory cells. This is the reason some medications work and others do not help individuals with asthma.

In addition, immunoglobulin E (abbreviated IgE) is a protein responsible for allergic responses and inflammation in the breath-

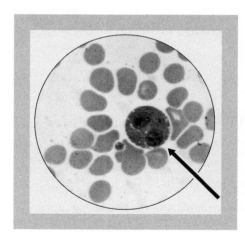

Figure 4.2 View from a microscope of an eosinophil shown by arrow surrounded by red blood cells. Eosinophils are specialized white blood cells. The two darker areas are the multilobed nuclei, and the dots are granules in the cytoplasma. (iStock.com/toeytoey2530)

ing tubes. IgE attaches to the walls of mast cells. When someone who is allergic inhales an allergen (e.g., pollen), the mast cells release numerous substances (called mediators) that cause narrowing of the airways (bronchoconstriction) and inflammation. Identifying individuals who have a high level of IgE is important because specific therapy is available that directly blocks its action.

Bronchoconstriction

A common feature of asthma is sudden tightening, or constriction, of the muscle that wraps around the breathing tubes. This is called bronchoconstriction and reduces the flow of air while exhaling. The common "triggers" that can cause narrowing of the breathing tubes are as follows:

Allergens (dust mites, grass, trees, pollen, etc.)
Irritants in the air (fumes, ozone, smoke, smog, etc.)
Exercise
Inhaling cold air
Stress

In general, the more inflamed the breathing tubes are, the greater the narrowing or constriction.

Figure 4.3 shows the changes in the breathing tubes in asthma. In addition to constriction, or tightening, of the smooth muscle, other factors can cause narrowing of the breathing tubes. One is edema or swelling of the wall of the breathing tubes. Another is mucus that is produced by glands that line the inside of the breathing tubes. This mucus usually consists of one or more types of inflammatory cells. A third is permanent damage to the breathing tubes. This can be due to scarring (called fibrosis) of the wall of the breathing tubes and thickening of the smooth muscle around the breathing tubes.

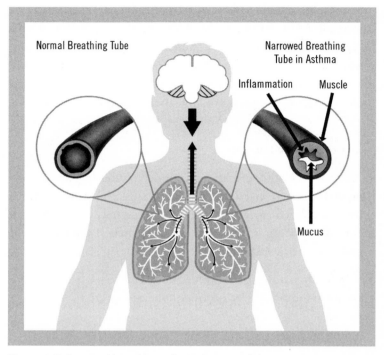

Figure 4.3 A normal breathing tube is shown on left. A narrowed breathing tube in someone with asthma is shown on right. Narrowing is due to three factors: smooth muscle that wraps around the breathing tube constricts or tightens, inflammation (redness and swelling), and mucus inside the breathing tube. (Based on iStock.com images from elenabs, kowalska-art, and stock_shoppe)

Symptoms

The main symptoms of asthma are as follows:

Shortness of breath: difficulty in breathing with activities
Wheezing: high-pitched whistling sounds when breathing out
Chest tightness: typically located in the center of the chest and
    may be described as a "squeezing" feeling
Cough: may be worse at night

These are due to redness/swelling (inflammation) and to narrowing (constriction) of the breathing tubes. Some individuals with asthma experience only one of these symptoms (e.g., cough), while others report all four of these problems. These symptoms can occur or worsen with exercise; upon exposure to smoke, animal dander, house dust mites, or pollen; when inhaling airborne irritants such as chemicals or perfumes; with a respiratory infection; when stress occurs; and with menstrual periods.

Asthma may be suspected by your doctor after looking at your medical history and after a physical examination. However, breathing tests, or pulmonary function tests (abbreviated PFTs), are required to diagnose asthma. Your health-care provider may order these tests if you report one or more of the symptoms listed above. You will usually undergo PFTs before and after inhaling albuterol, a quick-acting bronchodilator. The results will indicate whether there is narrowing of the breathing tubes (airflow obstruction), how bad it is (severity), and whether it improves, or reverses, with a bronchodilator. Sometimes, additional breathing tests are required to distinguish asthma from a vocal cord problem (called vocal cord dysfunction) and chronic obstructive pulmonary disease (COPD), which is discussed in chapter 5. Blood tests may be ordered to look for a specific type of inflammation such as eosinophils and IgE. Exhaled air can be analyzed to look for levels of nitric oxide, a marker of inflammation due to eosinophils.

Natural History

Natural history describes what usually happens over time with a particular illness. In asthma, the natural history is quite variable. In children with asthma, growth of the lung can be normal or reduced, and breathing tests (lung function) may decline. In those with asthma, symptoms may be intermittent (e.g., with a chest cold) or persistent (see table 4.1). In some adults, it appears that asthma may "morph" over time into chronic obstructive pulmonary disease (see chapter 5). With appropriate treatment, most individuals with asthma remain stable and lead a normal life.

Initial Assessment

Once the diagnosis of asthma has been made, it is important for you to work closely with your health-care provider in order to

identify "triggers" for asthma symptoms and inflammation (e.g., exposures to allergens or irritants);
identify other illnesses (called comorbidities) that may aggravate asthma, such as a sinus infection, nasal congestion, obstructive sleep apnea, and heartburn (acid reflux);
classify the severity of your asthma; and
learn more about asthma—in both discussions and use of written or online materials.

The severity of asthma is based on two considerations: how bad your asthma is (called impairment) and your risk of sudden worsening of asthma (called an exacerbation). Overall *impairment* includes frequency of symptoms (occasional or daily), nighttime awakenings (how often if at all), use of albuterol as rescue medication (how many times in a week), interference with daily activities, and results of breathing tests. *Risk* depends on how often you experienced a sudden worsening or "flare-up" of your asthma in the past year. Table 4.1 describes a simplified classification of asthma.

Asthma Control

The goals of therapy to achieve asthma control are to reduce impairment and to reduce the risk on worsening (exacerbation) of asthma. These are summarized in table 4.2.

Table 4.1 Simple classification of asthma

Mild intermittent	mild symptoms up to two days a week and up to two nights a week
Persistent	Mild: symptoms more than twice a week but no more than once in a single day
	Moderate: symptoms once a day and more than one night a week
	Severe: symptoms throughout the day on most days and frequently at night

Table 4.2 Goals of asthma control

Reduce impairment	Prevent symptoms (cough, shortness of breath, wheezing, and chest tightness)
	Require infrequent use of albuterol (ideally 0–2 times per week)
	Maintain normal or near-normal lung function (results of breathing tests)
	Maintain normal activities—at home, at work, and with exercise
Reduce risk of worsening or "flare-up"	Prevent recurrent worsening of asthma and need for emergency department visits
	Prevent loss of lung function (results of breathing tests)
	Provide best therapy with minimal or no side effects

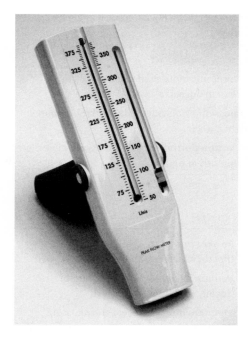

Figure 4.4 Peak flow meter. After you take a deep breath in, you put the mouthpiece into your mouth and blow out hard. A marker shows your peak flow value. This is a simple breathing test that can be done at home. (iStock.com/abalcazar)

Achievement of good asthma control depends on communication between you and your health-care provider. It also requires periodic monitoring and assessment of how you are doing. This should focus on your symptoms of asthma, results of your breathing tests (how your lungs are working), how often you are using albuterol or other rescue inhaler, and the effectiveness of medications that provide asthma control with hopefully few or no side effects. Your health-care provider should supply a written action plan in case you have breathing difficulty or experience worsening of your asthma.

Sometimes your health-care provider will recommend using a peak flow meter so you can measure how your lungs are working at home (figure 4.4). When asthma is first diagnosed, it is important to find your "personal best" peak flow for comparison at a later time. The highest number is considered your "best" when your asthma is well controlled. Typically, daily monitoring of your peak flow is useful to compare your breathing symptoms with how your lungs are working and when your asthma is not well controlled.

Environmental Control

Exposure to both allergens and irritants can cause immediate and chronic asthma symptoms. Therefore, it is important for you to avoid, or at least minimize, exposure if you are sensitive. Skin testing or blood tests may be helpful to identify specific things (allergens) that might "trigger" or aggravate your asthma. If you are sensitive to a pet in your home, the ideal treatment is to re-move the cat or dog from the home as all warm-blooded animals produce dander, urine, feces, and saliva that can cause allergic reactions. If it is not reasonable to remove the animal, then you should

keep the pet out of your bedroom;
keep the door to the bedroom closed;
remove upholstered furniture and carpets from the home,
    or isolate the pet from these items if possible; and
consider washing the pet weekly to remove large amounts of
    dander and dried saliva that would otherwise accumulate in
    the house.

Airborne irritants can also contribute to asthma symptoms and poor control. You should avoid tobacco smoke, smoke from fireplaces and woodburning stoves, and any odors (for example, perfumes and candle scents) that cause asthma symptoms. Some individuals with asthma are sensitive to aspirin and to sulfites used to preserve certain foods (shrimp and dried fruit), beer, and wine. Certainly, it is important to avoid these if you are sensitive. In general, certain foods (for example, nuts and shellfish) can cause itching, hives, and low blood pressure (anaphylaxis), but do not typically cause asthma symptoms.

If it is hot and humid where you live, use an air conditioner, which keeps it cool, lowers humidity, and reduces exposure to dust mites. If you live in a damp climate, consider using a dehumidifier. This will prevent or reduce mold spores. Clean your residence at least once a week. If you are likely to stir up dust, wear a mask or have someone else do the cleaning.

Medical Therapies (Pharmacotherapy)

Medical therapies used to treat asthma are classified as quick-acting bronchodilators and as long-term control medications. Quick-relief bronchodilators are used to treat sudden symptoms or worsening of asthma and are listed in table 4.3. The most widely used are called short-acting beta-agonists, of which albuterol sulfate is considered the first choice. Albuterol can also be used five to fifteen minutes before exercise to prevent asthma symptoms during exercise (called exercise-induced bronchoconstriction).

An alternative is a short-acting muscarinic antagonist called ipratropium bromide. It provides additive benefit to a short-acting beta-agonist because it works in a different way to relax the muscle that wraps around the outside of the breathing tubes. It is also used in those who do not tolerate short-acting beta-agonists. Albuterol sulfate and ipratropium bromide are available as a combination medication in a soft mist and in a solution used in a nebulizer.

Long-term control medications are used daily to achieve and maintain control for mild, moderate, or severe *persistent* asthma. Treatment is based on a step approach. "Step up" is used when asthma is not under good control. This means that higher doses or additional control medications are added. "Step down" is used when asthma control has been achieved and is stable. This means

Table 4.3 Quick-acting bronchodilators (last 4–6 hours) for treatment of asthma

GENERIC NAME	BRAND NAME	SUBSTANCE
Short-acting beta-agonists		
Albuterol sulfate	ProAir HFA	aerosol
	Proventil HFA	aerosol
	Ventolin HFA	aerosol
Albuterol sulfate		solution*
Levalbuterol tartrate	Xopenex HFA	aerosol and solution*
Pirbuterol	Maxair	aerosol
Short-acting muscarinic antagonists		
Ipratropium bromide	Atrovent HFA	aerosol and solution*
Combination		
Albuterol sulfate and	Combivent Respimat	soft mist
Ipratropium bromide	DuoNeb	solution*

*Solutions are used in nebulizers. All other medications are inhaled with a handheld device.

that doses can be reduced or control medications can be stopped one at a time.

The different types of these medications are listed in table 4.4. Inhaled corticosteroids are anti-inflammatory medications that are the most effective to improve asthma control. Studies show that inhaled corticosteroids reduce overall impairment and reduce the risk of worsening (an exacerbation) and are more effective than leukotriene modifiers—another class of an anti-inflammatory medication.

Leukotriene modifier medications interfere with a specific pathway that causes inflammation. These medications are alternative therapy to inhaled corticosteroids for those with mild persistent asthma. They are particularly effective in those with

Table 4.4 Long-term control medications for treatment of asthma

GENERIC NAME	BRAND NAME	SUBSTANCE
Inhaled corticosteroids		
Beclomethasone dipropionate	QVAR HFA	aerosol
Budesonide	Pulmicort Flexhaler	dry powder
Ciclesonide	Alvesco	aerosol
Mometasone	Asmanex HFA	aerosol
	Asmanex Twisthaler	dry powder
Fluticasone propionate	Flovent HFA	aerosol
	Flovent Diskus	dry powder
Fluticasone furoate	Annuity Ellipta	dry powder
Chromoglycates		
Cromolyn sodium*		solution†
Leukotriene modifiers		
Montelukast	Singulair (once daily)	tablet
Zafirlukast	Accolate (twice daily)	tablet
Zileuton	Zyflo (four times a day)	tablet
	Zyflo CR (twice daily)	tablet
Long-acting beta-agonists		
Formoterol fumarate	Foradil Aerolizer	aerosol
Salmeterol xinafoate	Serevent Diskus	dry powder
Long-acting muscarinic antagonists		
Tiotropium	Spiriva HandiHaler	dry powder
	Spiriva Respimat	soft mist

GENERIC NAME	BRAND NAME	SUBSTANCE
Combination Inhalers (inhaled corticosteroid and long-acting beta-agonist)		
TWICE DAILY		
Budesonide and formoterol	Symbicort	aerosol
Fluticasone propionate and salmeterol	Advair Diskus Advair HFA	dry powder aerosol
Mometasone and formoterol	Dulera	aerosol
ONCE DAILY		
Fluticasone furoate and vilanterol	Breo Ellipta	dry powder
Immunomodulators		
Omalizumab	Xolair	injection every 2–4 weeks
Mepolizumab	Nucala	injection monthly
Reslizumab	Cinqair	injection monthly

*Cromolyn is available as a dry-powder inhaler outside of the United States.
†Solutions are used in nebulizers. All other medications are inhaled with handheld device.

asthma who have nasal polyps and are sensitive to aspirin. In some individuals, leukotriene modifiers can be used in combination with inhaled corticosteroids. Leukotriene modifiers can also help with exercise-related asthma.

Long-acting beta-agonists (formoterol, brand name: Foradil; salmeterol, brand name: Serevent) are inhaled bronchodilators that, for twelve hours, relax the muscle that wraps around the breathing tubes. By relaxing the muscle, the breathing tubes can dilate, or enlarge, to allow greater flow of air and relieve breathing difficulty. These medicines are *not* used alone in the treatment of asthma but are rather used in combination with inhaled corticosteroids for those with moderate and severe persistent asthma. Combination medications that include an inhaled corticosteroid and a long-acting beta-agonist used once or twice daily are listed in table 4.4.

In addition, tiotropium (brand name: Spiriva) is a long-acting muscarinic antagonist bronchodilator that can be used as add-on therapy for those with asthma that is not adequately controlled with an inhaled corticosteroid and a long-acting beta-agonist bronchodilator. Oral sustained-release theophylline is a mild bronchodilator that is alternative therapy for persistent asthma. Its use has diminished over the years with the availability of newer and more effective asthma medications.

There are three immunomodulatory medications approved for the treatment of moderate to severe persistent asthma. These medications are generally used in those cases considered as *difficult to control* asthma. Each is administered as a shot (injection) under the skin (subcutaneous) either every two to four weeks (Xolair) or monthly (Nucala and Cinqair).

Omalizumab (brand name: Xolair) binds to IgE (anti-IgE) to prevent release of mediators that cause inflammation. It is used for those with moderate to severe persistent asthma who have allergies (usually shown by a positive skin test) and whose symptoms are not controlled with inhaled corticosteroids. Mepolizumab (brand name: Nucala) and reslizumab (brand name: Cinqair) are shots (injections) that block interleukin-5, which contributes to airway inflammation. These two medications help to prevent severe asthma attacks (exacerbations). They are used to treat those with severe asthma who have high blood levels of eosinophils (see figure 4.2).

All medications can cause possible side effects. Both mild and serious side effects of the different medications are described in table 4.5. The United States Food and Drug Administration requires a box warning for inhaled long-acting beta-agonists in

Table 4.5 Possible side effects of asthma medications

Beta-agonists
Mild: shakiness; increased heart rate; feeling nervous; trouble sleeping
Serious: irregular or fast heart rate; seizures; low potassium in the blood

Muscarinic antagonists
Mild: dryness of the mouth; cough; headache
Serious: difficulty urinating, especially in older men; glaucoma

Inhaled corticosteroids
Mild: hoarseness; yeast infection in the throat; bruising of the skin
Serious: cataracts; thinning of the bones (osteoporosis); pneumonia

Leukotriene modifiers
Mild: headache; abdominal pain; flu-like symptoms
Serious: difficulty sleeping; feeling sad; thoughts of suicide

Immunomodulators
You should review all possible side effects with your health-care provider

combination with an inhaled corticosteroid (Brand names: Advair, Breo, Dulera, and Symbicort) in treatment of those with asthma. In a study of 11,679 individuals with a history of a severe asthma exacerbation ("flare-up") in the past year, the fluticasone propionate and salmeterol combination was safe and reduced severe asthma "flare-ups" over the twenty-six weeks of the study.

Additional Therapies

ALLERGY SHOTS

Allergy shots have been used to reduce the body's immune response to specific allergens. They are usually given when there is a strong allergy component causing difficulty in obtaining good asthma control, especially when avoidance to exposure is not possible.

At first, shots are given once or twice a week for several months. The shot contains a tiny amount of whatever you are allergic to, such as pollen, pet dander, mold, dust mites, or bee venom. The dose is gradually increased until you reach a maintenance dose. Ideally, allergy shots will help relieve the allergic reactions that trigger asthma episodes, thereby improving how the lungs work and decreasing the need for asthma medications.

BRONCHIAL THERMOPLASTY

Bronchial thermoplasty is a treatment option for those with severe persistent asthma. It was approved by the United States Food and Drug Administration in 2010. A tube (called a bronchoscope) is placed into the mouth and then into the windpipe (trachea) and advanced into the breathing tubes. A smaller plastic tube is then placed through a channel inside the bronchoscope to deliver radiofrequency energy to the wall of the breathing tubes (airways) by heating the tissue and reducing the amount of smooth muscle present in the wall of the airways. The system delivers a series of ten-second temperature-controlled bursts that heat the lining of the breathing tubes to sixty-five degrees Celsius.

A full course of treatment is three separate bronchoscopies (passing a tube through the mouth into the breathing tubes), each approximately three weeks apart. One bronchoscopy is performed for each lower lobe of the lung, and the third is for both upper lobes. The benefits are improved asthma-related quality of life by reducing asthma attacks for at least five years. In addition, there are reductions in asthma attacks, visits to the emergency department, and hospitalizations for respiratory symptoms. The main risk is an expected brief increase in worsening of asthma symptoms in the period immediately following bronchial thermoplasty.

In the United States this treatment is primarily available at medical centers and large hospitals.

ALTERNATIVE TREATMENTS

Herbal and natural remedies have been used to help improve asthma symptoms. These include black seed (cumin), caffeine, choline (a nutrient), and pycnogenol (pine park extract). However, there is not enough evidence at the present to recommend these natural therapies. Other alternative treatments include yoga, acupuncture, an asthma diet, and biofeedback.

Referral to a Specialist

Most primary care providers are able to diagnose and treat asthma effectively to achieve good asthma control. However, some individuals have *difficult to control* asthma, and referral to a specialist may be appropriate. Both allergists (specialists in allergy and immunology) and pulmonologists (specialists in lung disease) have training and experience in asthma. The main reasons to see a specialist are as follows:

to confirm the diagnosis of asthma by breathing tests;
to identify triggers for inflammation in the breathing tubes (airways);
to evaluate for other conditions that might contribute to poor asthma control, such as allergies, sinusitis, acid reflux, allergic bronchopulmonary aspergillosis (a fungus in the breathing tubes), obesity, obstructive sleep apnea, and stress/depression;
to consider new treatment options; and
to discuss an asthma action plan if or when breathing worsens.

Key Points

> Asthma occurs when a person who has an increased risk (called genetic susceptibility) has an "injury" to the lungs. The "injury" may be an exposure to an allergen or a respiratory infection.

> Inflammation in the breathing tubes leads to narrowing (airway obstruction) and promotes constriction of the smooth muscle that wraps around breathing tubes (bronchoconstriction).
> These features lead to the symptoms of asthma: shortness of breath, wheezing, cough, and chest tightness.
> Asthma is classified by frequency of symptoms as intermittent or persistent. Persistent asthma may be mild, moderate, or severe.
> It is important to identify and avoid triggers to achieve good asthma control.
> Quick-acting inhaled bronchodilators are used for immediate relief of symptoms.
> Long-term control medications are used daily to achieve and maintain control of persistent asthma. Treatment is based on a step approach.
> Three injectable medications that directly affect the body's immune system are used in the treatment of moderate to severe persistent asthma. These medications are generally used in those considered as *difficult to control* asthma.
> It is important to follow an asthma action plan if your breathing gets worse. This includes monitoring your symptoms and possibly using a peak flow meter. Have albuterol inhaler readily available to use if needed.

References

Castro, Mario, et al. "Effectiveness and Safety of Bronchial Thermoplasty in the Treatment of Severe Asthma." *American Journal of Respiratory and Critical Care Medicine* 181 (2010): 116–24.

Chung, Kian Fan, et al. "International ERS/ATS Guidelines on Definition, Evaluation, and Treatment of Severe Asthma." *European Respiratory Journal* 43 (2014): 343–73.

Hanania, Nicola A., et al. "Omalizumab in Severe Allergic Asthma Inadequately Controlled with Standard Therapy." *Annals of Internal Medicine* 154 (2011): 573–82.

McGeachie, Michael J., et al. "Patterns of Growth and Decline in Lung Function in Persistent Childhood Asthma." *New England Journal of Medicine* 374 (2016): 1842–52.

National Heart, Lung, and Blood Institute. "Expert Panel Report 3: Guidelines for the Diagnosis and Management of Asthma." August 28, 2007. http://www.nhlbi.nih.gov/.

Stempel, David A., et al. "Serious Asthma Events with Fluticasone Plus Salmeterol versus Fluticasone Alone." *New England Journal of Medicine*, March 6, 2016. doi:10.1056/NEJMoa1511049 (Epub ahead of print).

(5)

Chronic Obstructive Pulmonary Disease

I wake up every day and I think, "I'm breathing! It's a good day."

Eve Ensler, activist and author of the *Vagina Monologues* (1953–)

Winning is the most important thing in my life, after breathing. Breathing first, winning next.

George Steinbrenner, former principal owner of New York Yankees (1930–2010)

In chronic obstructive pulmonary disease (COPD) there is narrowing of the breathing tubes (airways) that usually, but not always, gets worse over time. Cigarette smoking is the most common cause of COPD. However, inhaling dust, smoke, fumes, and fibers can also damage the lungs.

About 6 percent of those eighteen years of age or older in the United States have been diagnosed with COPD (figure 5.1). Utah has lowest rate at about 4 percent, and Kentucky has the highest rate at about 9 percent. Of United States adults aged forty to seventy-nine, about 14 percent have COPD. COPD is the third leading cause of death (after heart disease and cancer) in the United States. More women die of COPD each year than from breast cancer and diabetes combined.

COPD is both preventable and treatable. Generally, it can be prevented if you do not smoke cigarettes and do not inhale irritants in the air. Although there is no cure for COPD, there are many effective treatments available today. Inhaled medications can open the breathing tubes to make it easier to breathe and can prevent flare-ups (called exacerbations). Pulmonary rehabilitation

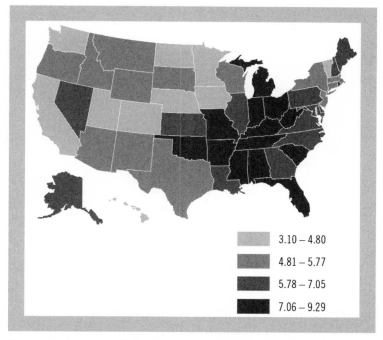

3.10 – 4.80
4.81 – 5.77
5.78 – 7.05
7.06 – 9.29

Figure 5.1 Map of the United States showing the percentage of adults in each state with a diagnosis of COPD. The darker-shaded states have the highest numbers. (iStock.com/HS3RUS)

provides many physical and psychological benefits (see chapter 8). Oxygen therapy relieves breathing difficulty and enables you to do physical activities for a longer time if you have a low oxygen level. Certain surgical procedures can "deflate" parts of the lungs and improve breathing if you have advanced emphysema (see chapter 9).

What Is COPD?

COPD is defined by Jørgen Vestbo and colleagues as a "preventable and treatable disease . . . characterized by persistent airflow

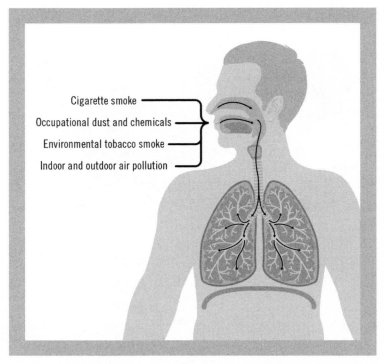

Figure 5.2 This diagram shows that the total burden of inhaling airborne irritants can injure the lungs in a susceptible individual. (Based on iStock. com images from elenabs and kowalska-art)

limitation that is usually progressive and associated with an enhanced chronic inflammatory response in the airways and the lung to noxious particles or gases" (349).

The definition means that smoking cigarettes and inhaling irritants (dust, chemicals, and air pollution) can cause redness and swelling (inflammation) in the breathing tubes and air sacs (alveoli) of the lungs (figure 5.2). However, COPD occurs in only one of five individuals who smoke a pack of cigarettes each day for at least twenty years. This suggests that there is a genetic (hereditary) susceptibility for individuals to the harmful effects of air-

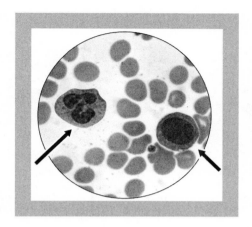

Figure 5.3 View from a microscope of a neutrophil on left and a lymphocyte on the right. The neutrophil has three lobules that form the nucleus. The lymphocyte has a large round structure in the middle called the nucleus. The other structures are red blood cells that are smaller than the neutrophil and lymphocyte. (iStock.com/ toeytoey2530)

borne irritants. Unfortunately, it is impossible to predict who will or will not "get" COPD if you smoke cigarettes or inhale "bad air." It is more likely that you will develop COPD if one or both of your parents had this condition.

In COPD, there are two major types of white blood cells that cause inflammation. These cells are neutrophils and CD8+ lymphocytes (figure 5.3). If inflammation occurs mainly in the breathing tubes, it is called chronic bronchitis. If inflammation and damage occur mainly in the air sacs, it is called emphysema. It is difficult to know or predict which areas of the lung might be affected by smoking and inhaling irritants. In chronic bronchitis, the major changes are that the glands in the breathing tubes produce mucus and the walls of the breathing tubes become thicker. These changes cause narrowing of the breathing tubes as shown in figure 5.4.

In emphysema, neutrophils release enzymes that digest and destroy elastic tissue of the air sacs. This digestive/destructive pro-

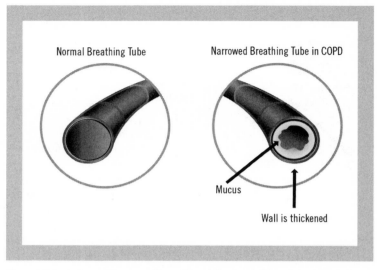

Figure 5.4 A view of a normal breathing tube (on left) and a narrowed breathing tube (on right) due to mucus and a thickened wall. The changes on the right reflect chronic bronchitis. (iStock.com/stock_shoppe)

cess is illustrated in figures 5.5 and 5.6. This process leads to loss of the elasticity of the lung and reduces the pressure that helps to exhale air out of the lungs.

These three factors—mucus, thickening of the walls of the tubes, and destruction of the air sacs—along with constriction, or tightening, of the muscle that wraps around the breathing tubes reduce the flow of air out of the breathing tubes. This is called air-flow obstruction.

Whether you develop chronic bronchitis, emphysema, or a combination of the two depends on your body's response to the harmful effects of smoking cigarettes or inhaling airborne irritants. Chronic bronchitis is usually defined as cough that produces mucus on most days for at least three months for two years in a row.

In emphysema, air is trapped in the lungs as a result of the

Figure 5.5 Process of how smoking cigarettes causes an increase in neutrophils, inflammatory white blood cells. Neutrophils release enzymes called proteinases that digest and destroy elastin tissue in the air sacs. This leads to emphysema. (LeftRightCreative)

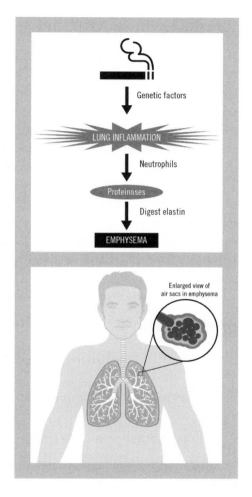

Figure 5.6 A view of damaged and enlarged air sacs is shown on the right. (Based on iStock.com images from elenabs and kowalska-art)

destruction of the air sacs. It comes from the Greek word that means "puff up." Many of those with COPD have components of both chronic bronchitis and emphysema. Shortness of breath, or breathing difficulty, with daily activities is the most common complaint of having COPD. Coughing and wheezing may also occur.

The Diagnosis of COPD

You may have been told that you have COPD by a health-care provider because you reported shortness of breath or a daily cough along with a history of smoking cigarettes. However, breathing tests, also called pulmonary function tests (PFTs), are required to diagnose COPD. It is necessary to demonstrate airflow obstruction as shown in figure 5.7. Airflow obstruction means there is reduced flow of air out of the lungs when you exhale.

Sometimes, your health-care provider may request that you perform breathing tests before and after inhaling albuterol, a quick-acting bronchodilator. The results will indicate whether there is narrowing of the breathing tubes (airflow obstruction), how bad it is (severity), and whether it improves, or reverses, with a bronchodilator.

In summary, the diagnosis of COPD depends on three factors:

symptoms such as shortness of breath with activities or chronic cough;

a history of smoking cigarettes or inhaling irritants in the air; and

airflow obstruction on breathing tests.

Alpha-1 Antitrypsin Deficiency

Alpha-1 antitrypsin (abbreviated Alpha-1) is a protein made in the liver that is released into the blood before traveling to the lungs. The Alpha-1 protein protects the lung from damage. In Alpha-1 deficiency, some of the protein is blocked in the liver and does not reach the lungs. As a result, there is loss of the normal protective effects due to the low level of Alpha-1 protein in the lungs. The lungs are then more susceptible to injury or damage from smoking cigarettes or inhaling irritants in the air. Alpha-1 deficiency is

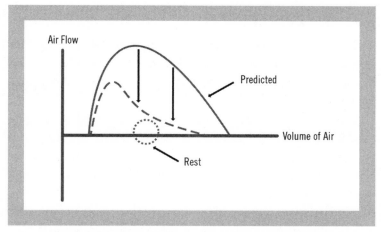

Figure 5.7 The predicted flow of air during exhalation in a healthy person is shown in the nonbroken line. The flow of air during exhalation in someone who has COPD is shown in the dashed curve. The downward arrows show reduced airflow compared to normal. (LeftRightCreative)

a hereditary form of emphysema and is most common among Europeans and North Americans of European descent.

Alpha-1 deficiency should be suspected in anyone who has COPD, particularly if the disease occurs at an early age (under forty-five years of age); emphysema is evident in the lower parts of the lungs on chest x-ray or CT scan; and you have unexplained liver disease.

The condition is diagnosed by measuring the Alpha-1 protein in the blood. It is recommended that everyone who has COPD be tested for Alpha-1 deficiency. It is important to make the diagnosis for two main reasons: specific therapy is available to treat Alpha-1 related lung disease, and family members should be informed so that they can be tested.

Treatment for Alpha-1 deficiency is called augmentation therapy. It consists of the Alpha-1 protein obtained from the blood of healthy human donors. This solution is given once a week intra-venously in order to increase the level of Alpha-1 protein in the lungs. This treatment should protect the lungs from any further destruction as long as the person does not smoke. Although aug-mentation therapy cannot repair damaged lung tissue, the goal is to prevent further destruction of the lungs.

There are four augmentation products approved by the U.S. Food and Drug Administration. The brand names of these prod-ucts are Aralast NP; Glassia, Prolastin-C; and Zemaira. The in-fusions are typically given by a health-care professional in the home, at a physician's office, or at an infusion center in a hospital. Health insurance companies often determine where the infusion is given. It is recommended that all those receiving augmentation therapy be immunized for hepatitis A and B to reduce the risk of liver injury.

Natural History

In healthy individuals, lung function as measured by breath-ing tests gets worse (declines) slowly after the age of fifty. This is due to aging as the lung loses elasticity. For those with COPD, breathing tests generally decline faster than normal over time. This belief was based on results of a study from the United King-dom published in 1976. However, recent studies reveal that this is not completely accurate. Rather, there are two different pathways for those who have COPD: in some individuals there is a slow but steady decline in breathing tests that is greater than expected with aging, and in others breathing tests remain fairly stable.

These results show that the natural history of COPD is variable. It is important to understand that it is impossible to predict the course of COPD for any individual. However, if you continue to smoke cigarettes, there is strong evidence that your lung func-tion will get worse faster than if you did not smoke. Some studies suggest that long-acting inhaled bronchodilators and inhaled corticosteroid medications may stabilize the course of COPD.

Differences between Men and Women

For the first time, in the year 2000, more women in the United States died of COPD than men. Although smoking tobacco products is the biggest risk factor for developing COPD, women who live in developing countries are at risk due to inhaling smoke and other irritants from cooking and heating with coal and wood. For the same level of lung function (breathing test results), women report more breathlessness and have lower scores for quality of life. Women with COPD have higher levels of anxiety and depression than men, which may aggravate the experience of breathing discomfort. Men and women appear to respond differently to cigarette smoking as chronic bronchitis is more common in women, whereas emphysema is more common in men.

An Exacerbation of COPD

The word "exacerbation" means a worsening. An exacerbation of COPD is commonly called a "flare-up" as the individual has an increase in breathing difficulty, an increase in coughing and in coughing up mucus, and a change in color of the mucus (from clear to yellow or green). There are several risk factors for having a COPD exacerbation. These include the following:

older age;
a daily cough that produces mucus (called chronic bronchitis);
air pollution;
other medical conditions such as heartburn (gastroesophageal
    reflux disease), diabetes, or heart disease; and
previous COPD exacerbations.

Your risk of having another exacerbation depends on the number of flare-ups that you had in the past year. If you had only one or no flare-ups, the risk is low; for two or more flare-ups, the risk is high.

There are several different causes of a COPD flare-up. In general, most exacerbations are due to a chest infection that may be bacterial or viral. Typically, with a bacterial infection, the person coughs up yellow or green mucus; with a viral infection, the mucus is usually clear or gray. The infection is called *acute bronchitis* if it involves the breathing tubes and is called *pneumonia* if it involves the air sacs.

About 20–30 percent of exacerbations are related to environmental conditions, especially air pollution. Smog is produced by factories; exhaust from cars, buses, and trucks; and emissions from furnaces that become "trapped" in the air. This may occur with humid weather when there is little air movement outdoors. Some people describe the air as being "heavy," making it more difficult to breathe. Air pollutants irritate the breathing tubes and cause inflammation and bronchoconstriction. Heart failure and blood clots that travel to the lungs (called pulmonary embolism) may cause breathing problems that mimic an exacerbation.

Initial Assessment

Once the diagnosis has been made, it is recommended that your health-care provider assess your COPD based on symptoms (mainly shortness of breath) and risk of an exacerbation. Four different groups can be identified, as shown in table 5.1.

Your health-care provider should also identify other illnesses (called comorbidities) that may affect your COPD. These include bronchiectasis, obstructive sleep apnea, heart disease, and acid reflux (called gastroesophageal reflux disease).

Table 5.1 Simple classification of COPD

GROUP	SYMPTOMS	RISK OF AN EXACERBATION
A	Few	Low
B	More	Low
C	Few	High
D	More	High

Table 5.2 Goals of treating COPD

Reduce symptoms
> Relieve symptoms (shortness of breath, cough, and wheezing)
> Improve exercise tolerance
> Improve health status

Reduce risk
> Prevent disease progression
> Prevent exacerbations
> Reduce mortality

Goals of Therapy

The goals of therapy for those with COPD are summarized in table 5.2.

Smoking Cessation

The most important action is to stop smoking and to avoid inhaling dust, smoke, fumes, and other irritants in the air. By quitting smoking, you not only prevent further damage to your lungs but also lower your chances of getting heart disease or lung cancer and reduce the possibility of thinning of the bones (osteoporosis).

To get started, you should think about what you like and what you do not like about smoking. For example, some people find that smoking helps deal with stress. You should set a quit date and tell others that you plan to quit. There are numerous resources, both local hospitals and national organizations, available to help you quit smoking permanently.

About 10 percent of those who quit smoking do it "cold turkey." For others, nicotine-replacement products are available to help with nicotine withdrawal (irritability, anxiety, difficulty concentrating, and difficulty sleeping). Products include nicotine patches, gum, sprays, and lozenges that enable nicotine to enter via the blood instead of through smoking a cigarette. Prescription medications are available to reduce the desire to smoke. These include bupropion (brand name: Wellbutrin) and varenicline (brand name: Chantix). You should discuss with your health-care provider whether these treatments are appropriate for you.

Lifestyle changes can also be helpful to quit smoking. You should stay away from family members or friends when they smoke. For example, ask these people to smoke outside rather than indoors. Keep oral substitutes nearby, such as sugarless gum or carrots, to deal with cravings. Consider learning relaxation techniques to reduce stress, and start to exercise to improve health and fitness. You may also wish to join a support program or participate in group counseling. For some individuals, hypnosis and acupuncture have been helpful to quit smoking.

Medical Therapies (Pharmacotherapy)

Some inhaled medications used to treat those with COPD are also used to treat asthma. For example, quick-relief bronchodilators relieve the sudden onset of shortness of breath. These are listed in table 4.4 of chapter 4 on asthma. The most widely used is albuterol sulfate, a short-acting beta-agonist. An alternative is ipratropium bromide, a short-acting muscarinic antagonist. The combination of albuterol sulfate and ipratropium bromide is available in a soft mist and in a solution for use in a nebulizer.

Table 5.3 Long-acting bronchodilators for treatment of COPD

GENERIC NAME	BRAND NAME	SUBSTANCE
Long-acting beta-agonists		
TWICE DAILY		
Arformoterol tartate	Brovana	solution*
Formoterol fumarate	Perforomist	solution*
Formoterol fumarate	Foradil Aerolizer	aerosol
Salmeterol xinafoate	Serevent Diskus	dry powder
ONCE DAILY		
Indacaterol	Arcapta Neohaler	dry powder
Olodaterol	Striverdi Respimat	soft mist
Long-acting muscarinic antagonists		
TWICE DAILY		
Aclidinium	Tudorza Pressair	dry powder
Glycopyrrolate	Seebri Neohaler†	dry powder
ONCE DAILY		
Tiotropium	Spiriva HandiHaler	dry powder
	Spiriva Respimat	soft mist
Umeclidinium	Incruse Ellipta	dry powder

*Solutions are used in nebulizers. All other medications are inhaled with handheld device.
†Used in a different dose once daily outside of the United States.

Long-acting inhaled bronchodilators are maintenance therapies to open the breathing tubes, "deflate" the lungs, and make it easier to breathe. The two different types of bronchodilators — long-acting beta-agonists and long-acting muscarinic antagonists — are often used together because they work in different ways (table 5.3). By relaxing the muscle that wraps around the breathing tubes, these medications allow greater flow of air during exhalation and enable the lungs to empty more air. This helps to relieve breathing

Table 5.4 Long-acting combination medications
for treatment of COPD

GENERIC NAME	BRAND NAME	SUBSTANCE
Inhaled long-acting beta-agonist and long-acting muscarinic antagonist		
TWICE DAILY		
Indacaterol and glycopyrrolate	Utibron Neohaler*	dry powder
Formoterol and glycopyrrolate	Bevespi Aerosphere	aerosol
ONCE DAILY		
Vilanterol and umeclidinium	Anoro Ellipta	dry powder
Olodaterol and tiotropium	Stiolto Respimat	soft mist
Inhaled corticosteroid and long-acting beta-agonist		
TWICE DAILY		
Budesonide and formoterol	Symbicort	aerosol
Fluticasone propionate and salmeterol	Advair Diskus	dry powder
	Advair HFA	aerosol
ONCE DAILY		
Fluticasone furoate and vilanterol	Breo Ellipta	dry powder

*Used in different doses once daily outside of the United States.

difficulty. These long-acting bronchodilators last for either twelve (used twice daily) or twenty-four (used once daily) hours.

Combination products are available that include two different types of medications in a single inhaler. These combinations are listed in table 5.4. Studies show that the combination of two bronchodilators in a single device is more effective in opening the breathing tubes and allowing individuals to breathe easier compared with only one bronchodilator. This approach is also convenient for those with COPD compared with using two different inhaler devices.

Inhaled corticosteroids are anti-inflammatory medications that help to reduce the risk of an exacerbation of COPD. Inhaled corticosteroids are approved for use in those with COPD in combination with a long-acting beta-agonist.

All medications can cause possible side effects. Both mild and serious side effects of the different medications are as follows:

BETA-AGONISTS

Mild: shakiness; increased heart rate; feeling nervous; trouble sleeping

Serious: irregular or fast heart rate; seizures; low potassium in the blood

MUSCARINIC ANTAGONISTS

Mild: dryness of the mouth; cough; headache

Serious: difficulty urinating, especially in older men; glaucoma

INHALED CORTICOSTEROIDS

Mild: hoarseness; yeast infection in the throat; bruising of the skin

Serious: cataracts; thinning of the bones (osteoporosis); pneumonia

COPD Action Plan

An action plan is what to do in case you experience worsening or a flare-up of your breathing. This information should be written down and easy to find. Here is a simple COPD action plan:

1 If you are more short of breath, use albuterol sulfate or ipratropium bromide every two to four hours as needed.
2 If you cough up yellow or green mucus, call or see your healthcare provider to ask if an antibiotic is appropriate.
3 If use of albuterol sulfate or ipratropium bromide does not help improve your breathing difficulty, call or see your healthcare provider to ask if prednisone is appropriate.

4 If you cannot speak in full sentences or cannot fall asleep at night because of breathing difficulty, call or see your health-care provider, go to an urgent care center, or go to the nearest emergency department.

Treatment of an exacerbation starts with increased use of one or two short-acting inhaled bronchodilators. These are albuterol (brand names: ProAir, Proventil, and Ventolin) and ipratropium (brand name: Atrovent). These medications are available in inhalers or in solutions delivered with a nebulizer.

An antibiotic is usually prescribed if you have a bacterial infection (coughing up yellow or green mucus). For most viral infections, there are no effective antibiotics. However, antiviral drugs are available to treat the flu (influenza) virus if it is diagnosed within forty-eight hours of start of symptoms. Oseltamivir (brand name: Tamiflu) is prescribed for five days and can lessen symptoms and shorten the time you are sick by one or two days. It can also prevent serious flu complications, such as pneumonia.

If the exacerbation causes you to feel more short of breath, a corticosteroid (often called a steroid) is frequently prescribed. It reduces inflammation in the breathing tubes and improves the flow of air. The usual steroid medication is a pill called prednisone if you are treated at home; an intravenous corticosteroid is commonly given if you are admitted to the hospital. Oxygen therapy may be required if the exacerbation lowers your blood oxygen level.

It is hard to predict how long the shortness of breath, coughing, and wheezing of an exacerbation will last. For some, it may last one or more weeks. For others, it may take one or more months to recover completely. It is most important that you start to feel better within a few days of starting treatment. If not, you should contact your health-care provider.

Preventing an Exacerbation

There are many strategies to reduce the chances of you having an exacerbation. Most important, you should not smoke and should avoid inhaling irritants in the air. Vaccinations for the flu and for the most common bacteria that causes pneumonia (called Streptococcus pneumoniae) reduce the risk of an exacerbation occurring. Participation in pulmonary rehabilitation (see chapter 8) provides many benefits including helping to prevent a COPD exacerbation.

Four medications are approved by the U.S. Food and Drug Administration to reduce the risk of an exacerbations of COPD. These include

tiotropium (brand name: Spiriva), an inhaled long-acting, once-daily bronchodilator;

fluticasone propionate and salmeterol (brand name: Advair), an inhaled long-acting, twice-daily combination of a corticosteroid and a long-acting bronchodilator;

fluticasone furoate and vilanterol (brand name: Breo), an inhaled long-acting, once-daily combination of a corticosteroid and a long-acting bronchodilator; and

roflumilast (brand name: Daliresp), a once-daily pill.

The first three inhaled medications also open the airways and make it easier to breathe because they contain a bronchodilator. Roflumilast is approved for those with COPD who have chronic bronchitis, have severe COPD based on results of breathing tests, and have a history of frequent exacerbations. Also, the antibiotic azithromycin may be prescribed three times a week for those with a history of exacerbations in addition to the use of one or more of the medications listed above. As with all medications, you should discuss expected benefits along with possible side effects with your health-care provider.

Referral to a Specialist

Most primary care providers are able to diagnose and treat COPD. However, some individuals with COPD may have persistent problems, especially shortness of breath and recurrent chest infections leading to exacerbations. In such situations, referral to a specialist in lung disease (pulmonologist) may be appropriate. Some of the reasons to see a pulmonologist are as follows:

to confirm the diagnosis of COPD;
to test for Alpha-1 deficiency;
to evaluate for other conditions that might contribute to
    persistent symptoms;
to consider new treatments or different medications;
to discuss a COPD action plan if or when breathing worsens; and
to provide education about the disease.

Asthma-COPD Overlap Syndrome

Most health-care providers can determine whether you have asthma or COPD. Asthma usually occurs at an early age, is often associated with allergies, and has a good response to inhaled therapies. COPD is typically diagnosed after the age of forty, is usually associated with cigarette smoking, and tends to slowly get worse.

It is estimated that 10 to 20 percent of those with COPD also have features of asthma. This is called the asthma-COPD overlap syndrome (ACOS). In ACOS, there is persistent narrowing of the breathing tubes (airflow obstruction) with features of both asthma and COPD. Two typical examples are as follows: a young individual with asthma may have features of COPD due to smoking or scarring of the breathing tubes (airway remodeling); and a person with COPD may have features of asthma due to allergies.

It appears that those with ACOS experience more frequent and severe exacerbations or flare-ups. At the present time, health-care providers often prescribe medications for those with ACOS that treat both asthma and COPD. This approach includes use of inhaled beta-agonist and muscarinic antagonist bronchodilators as well as inhaled corticosteroids. This is commonly called "triple therapy."

Key Points

> COPD is preventable and treatable.
> About one out of five adults who smoke a pack of cigarettes each day for twenty or more years develops COPD.
> In COPD there is narrowing of the breathing tubes that causes airflow obstruction.
> Chronic bronchitis and emphysema are the two major types of COPD.
> The diagnosis of COPD depends on three factors:
  1 a history of smoking cigarettes or inhaling irritants in the air;
  2 shortness of breath or daily cough; and
  3 breathing tests that show narrowing of the breathing tubes (airways obstruction).
> All individuals diagnosed with COPD should be tested for Alpha-1 antitrypsin deficiency, an inherited form of emphysema.
> A COPD exacerbation is a flare-up with one or more of the following symptoms: an increase in breathing difficulty, an increase in coughing, coughing up more mucus, or a change in color of the mucus.
> Both short- and long-acting inhaled bronchodilators are available to reduce shortness of breath and to improve quality of life.

> Medications are available that reduce the risk of an exacerbation or flare-up of COPD.
> A written action plan is important in case of a flare-up of COPD.

References

Batemen, Eric D., et al. "Recent Advances in COPD Disease Management with Fixed-Dose Long-Acting Combination Therapies." *Expert Review of Respiratory Medicine* 8 (2014): 357–79.

COPD Foundation. http://www.copdfoundation.org/.

donaldmahler.com (website with information that positively affects the daily lives of those with COPD and their families).

Mahler, Donald A. *COPD: Answers to Your Questions*. Minneapolis: Two Harbors Press, 2015.

Qaseem, Amir, et al. "Diagnosis and Management of Stable Chronic Obstructive Pulmonary Disease: A Clinical Practice Guideline Update from the American College of Physicians, American College of Chest Physicians, American Thoracic Society, and European Respiratory Society." *Annals of Internal Medicine* 155 (2011): 179–91.

Vestbo, Jørgen, et al. "Global Strategy for the Diagnosis, Management, and Prevention of Chronic Obstructive Pulmonary Disease: GOLD Executive Summary." *American Journal of Respiratory and Critical Care Medicine* 187 (2013): 347–65.

(6)

Correct Inhaler Use

Most diseases are treated with pills. However, inhaling one or more medications is the main approach for the treatment of those with asthma and chronic obstructive pulminary disease (COPD). There are two types of inhaled medications for both asthma and COPD that work in different ways:

bronchodilators: relax the smooth muscle that wraps around the breathing tubes; and
corticosteroids: reduce inflammation (swelling and redness) in the lining of the breathing tubes.

To be effective, the medication needs to be inhaled into the mouth, make a sharp downward turn while passing through the throat, go between the vocal cords, enter the windpipe (trachea), and then travel through large breathing tubes (bronchi) before reaching the lower breathing tubes (bronchioles; figure 6.1).

The ability of an individual to inhale a medication deep into the lungs depends on correct technique, including adequate flow of air while breathing in. The major advantage of inhaling a medication is that it acts directly in the lungs. Only a minimal amount of medication is absorbed and reaches other parts of the body. This approach reduces possible side effects compared with swallowing a pill, when the medication is absorbed in the blood stream and then distributed throughout the body.

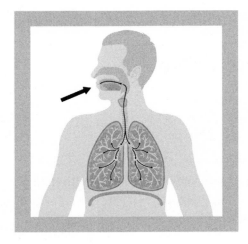

Figure 6.1 Pathway of inhaled medication reaching the lower breathing tubes. (Based on iStock.com images from elenabs and kowalska-art)

Delivery Systems

There are four different delivery systems for inhaled medications:

a pressurized metered-dose inhaler (pMDI) releases an aerosol (spray);

a propellant-free spring-loaded device (called Respimat) releases a fine mist;

a powder is inhaled from a dry-powder inhaler (DPI); and

a liquid is placed in a container (cup) attached to a nebulizer machine.

It is important for you to understand these different delivery systems in order to achieve the expected benefits.

Studies show that many individuals with asthma and COPD do not use their inhaler devices correctly. A recent report highlighted the most frequent inhaler errors. The systematic review included a total of 54,354 individuals who were directly observed for correct inhaler technique by trained personnel. For pMDI use, the three most frequent errors were no breath hold after inhaling (46 percent);

poor coordination for activating the inhaler and inhaling the
    aerosol (45 percent); and

incorrect speed or depth of inhaling (44 percent).

For DPI use, the three most frequent errors were not exhaling
completely before inhaling the powder (46 percent); no breath
hold after inhaling (37 percent); and incorrect preparation of the
DPI (28 percent). This information demonstrates that incorrect
inhaler technique is common. More importantly, poor technique
is associated with higher rates of being hospitalized and more frequent visits to the emergency department compared with correct
inhaler use in those with COPD.

Correct Inhaler Techniques

The following step-by-step instructions describe correct inhaling techniques. Different approaches are required for each type
of delivery systems. *It is important to remember that you need to be
able to inhale the medication deep into the breathing tubes for the
medication to work.*

PRESSURIZED METERED-DOSE INHALER

This device releases a specific amount of water droplets mixed
with air through an aerosol. The pressurized canister is held inside a plastic holder with a mouthpiece attached at one end (figure
6.2). When you push the canister down, the aerosol medication is
released under pressure.

With correct inhalation technique, only about 10 percent of the
aerosol that comes out of the inhaler reaches the lower breathing
tubes. Some of the medication hits the tongue and the throat.
This makes it very important to use the pMDI correctly.

Both "open-mouth" and "closed-mouth" techniques are used

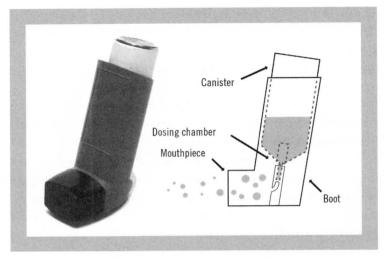

Figure 6.2 Example of a pressurized metered-dose inhaler. (iStock.com/markhicksphotography)

for inhaling medication from a pMDI. With the open-mouth technique, keep the inhaler about two fingers from the lips. With the closed-mouth technique, place the mouthpiece of the inhaler into your mouth. You should review each step before using your pMDI medication to make sure you are inhaling correctly. If you do not follow these instructions, even less of the medication will reach your lower breathing tubes. If you are not sure that you are using the pMDI according to instructions, you should ask your healthcare provider or nurse to watch you when you inhale medication from the device.

INSTRUCTIONS FOR USING A PRESSURIZED METERED-DOSE INHALER

1 Shake the pMDI vigorously for a few seconds.
2 Take the cap off of the mouthpiece.
3 Hold the pMDI upright with your index finger on the top of the canister and your thumb at the bottom of the inhaler.

4   Slowly breathe out all of the air from your lungs.

5   Place the pMDI about two fingers in front of your mouth (called open-mouth technique), *or* place the mouthpiece inside your mouth and close your lips around the mouthpiece (called closed-mouth technique).

6   As you start to breathe in *slowly* through your mouth, press down on the top of the canister with your index finger to release the medication.

7   Breathe in with a *slow and steady* effort until you fill your lungs with air.

8   Hold your breath for ten seconds or for as long as possible. This allows the aerosol to reach the lower breathing tubes.

9   Wait fifteen to thirty seconds, and then repeat steps 4 to 8 to inhale another dose of the medication.

10   If the medication contains an inhaled corticosteroid, you should rinse your mouth with water and spit out the water.

Many pMDIs have a dose counter that indicates the number of puffs remaining in the device.

If your pMDI is new, or if it has not been used in two weeks, you need to prime the inhaler as described below. Priming enables you to get the full dose of the inhaled medication. Each pharmaceutical company provides recommendations for priming the particular pMDI.

PRIMING YOUR PRESSURIZED
METERED-DOSE INHALER

1   Shake the pMDI vigorously for a few seconds.

2   Take the cap off of the mouthpiece.

3   Press down on the canister, and spray the aerosol away from you three to four times into the air. This will waste three to four puffs.

4   The pMDI is now ready for use.

The pMDI should be cleaned regularly every one to two weeks to prevent medication buildup and blockage at the opening. Remove the canister and cap from the mouthpiece. Run warm tap water through the top and bottom of the plastic mouthpiece for thirty to sixty seconds. Then, shake off excess water and allow the mouthpiece to dry (overnight is recommended).

USING A SPACER WITH A pMDI

A spacer offers several advantages for using a pMDI (figure 6.3). First, it removes any difficulty with coordinating activation of the pMDI and inhaling the medication. Second, it helps the larger aerosol particles evaporate so there are smaller particles in the spacer that can reach deeper into the breathing tubes. Third, it makes it easier to take a slow inhalation, which is necessary for the aerosol spray to make the sharp turn from the back of the mouth down to the windpipe (trachea) and into the breathing tubes.

A spacer should be used with a pMDI if you have difficulty with coordination or if you are using a pMDI that contains an inhaled corticosteroid. It is important to understand that you need to start inhaling within three seconds of pressing down (actuating) the pMDI. This is so that the aerosol particles remain suspended in the spacer for less than ten seconds. A spacer will also decrease the amount of aerosol deposited in the mouth and throat. You should ask your health-care provider whether a spacer in necessary.

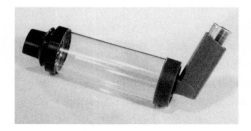

Figure 6.3 Example of a spacer and pMDI. (iStock. com/davidf)

INSTRUCTIONS FOR USING A PRESSURIZED
METERED-DOSE INHALER WITH A SPACER

1   Shake the pMDI vigorously for a few seconds.
2   Take the cap off of the mouthpiece.
3   Place the pMDI into the end of the spacer.
4   Breathe out normally away from the spacer (do not exhale into the spacer).
5   Put your mouth around the mouthpiece of the spacer and close your lips.
6   Press down on the top of the pMDI canister with your index finger to release the aerosol spray into the spacer.
7   Within three seconds of pressing down on the canister, breathe in *slowly* until you have filled your lungs with air.
8   If you hear a whistle sound, you are breathing in too fast.
9   Hold your breath for ten seconds or for as long as possible. This allows the aerosol to reach the lower airways.
10 Wait fifteen to thirty seconds, and then repeat to inhale another dose of the medication.
11 If the medication contains an inhaled corticosteroid, you should rinse your mouth with water and spit out the water.

Most manufacturers of spacers recommend that the device be cleaned every one to two weeks. Wash the spacer with warm water and dishwashing detergent. Washing with water alone causes an electrostatic charge to develop that reduces the effectiveness of the spacer. After washing, air-dry the spacer before the next use. You should *not* wipe or rub the inner surface of the spacer as this adds to the surface charge of the spacer.

USING THE RESPIMAT INHALER

The Respimat device delivers a "soft mist" through a nozzle. Twisting the base 180 degrees (one-half turn) compresses a spring and builds up mechanical power. The instructions for using this device are different from for a pMDI. Use of the Respimat is a three-step process summarized by T-O-P.

T Turn the plastic base one-half of a turn until you hear a click.
O Open the plastic cap that covers the mouthpiece. Breathe out slowly, and then place your lips around the end of the mouthpiece.
P Press the black release button while taking a slow and steady breath in, and continue to breathe in for as long as possible. Then, hold your breath for ten seconds or for as long as possible.

You should repeat the T-O-P steps for a second dose of tiotropium (brand name: Spiriva), olodaterol (brand name: Striverdi), and tiotropium-olodaterol combination (brand name: Stiolto). Only one inhalation (puff) is the standard dose for albuterol-ipratropium combination (brand name: Combivent). Just as with a pMDI, the Respimat device should be primed three to four times before initial use.

USING A DRY-POWDER INHALER

A dry-powder inhaler (DPI) contains a medication in a dry-powder form. The dry powder is either held in a capsule to be loaded into the device with each use (single-dose devices) or stored in powder packets inside the device (multiple-dose devices). The force of your inhalation breaks up the powder into small particles that can reach the lower breathing tubes.

A DPI is "breath actuated," which means that no coordination is required between activating the device and inhaling the medication. All DPIs have some internal resistance so that you need to breathe in *hard and fast* to break up the powder into small particles. This requires that you have an adequate inspiratory flow (the force of breathing in). If you do not breathe in hard and fast, a lot of the medication will be deposited in your mouth and throat. You should discuss the correct inhalation technique of your DPI with your health-care provider or the nurse because each DPI has slightly different instructions for use.

Instructions for using a DPI depend on the device. You should ask your health-care provider or review the package insert for specific information. The following instructions summarize general use of a DPI.

INSTRUCTIONS FOR USING A DRY-POWDER INHALER

1 For single-use devices, load the capsule into the device.
2 For multiple-use devices, press a lever, turn the base, or push down on the cover.
3 Slowly breathe out all of the air from your lungs (not into the mouthpiece).
4 Place the mouthpiece between your front teeth, and close your lips around it.
5 Breathe in *hard and fast* over two to three seconds.
6 Hold your breath for ten seconds or for as long as possible. This allows the powder particles to reach the lower airways.

USING A NEBULIZER

A fourth delivery system is placing a liquid medication into a container (cup) that is connected to a nebulizer. A nebulizer machine uses oxygen, compressed air, or ultrasonic power to break up the liquid medication into a mist that can be inhaled from a mouthpiece connected by tubing to the nebulizer (figure 6.4). The major components are the compressor, tubing, nebulizer cup for the medication, and mouthpiece.

Inhaling a medication from a nebulizer is recommended if you are unable to use the pMDI, Respimat, or DPI because of a physical or cognitive problem, such as arthritis of the fingers or hand, a stroke, or dementia;

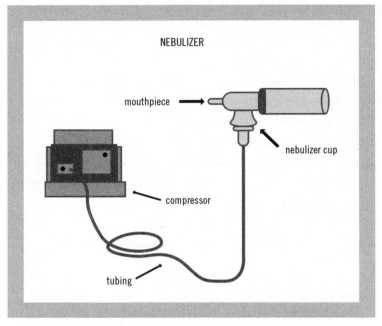

Figure 6.4 Nebulizer machine for breaking up a liquid medication into a mist. (LeftRightCreative)

have difficulty coordinating your breathing and holding your breath;

do not achieve the expected benefits with use of one or more inhalers despite using correct technique; or

do not have enough force when breathing in to pull the powder out of the DPI device.

One of the major advantages of using a nebulized medication is that you *breathe in and out normally* and do not need any special breathing technique required with other delivery systems (pMDI, Respimat, or DPI). However, it may take up to ten minutes to inhale medication from a nebulizer, and the system requires cleaning.

Your health-care provider can order a nebulizer machine and appropriate medications. A nurse, respiratory therapist, or some-one who works for a home-care company can instruct you about how to use the nebulizer with the medications and how to clean the system. The nebulizer and medications may also be obtained at a pharmacy. The following information describes how to inhale the aerosol medication from a nebulizer. There are portable nebu-lizers with the option of a rechargeable battery so that you are able to take it with you when you travel. A car adapter may also be used to power the device.

INSTRUCTIONS FOR USING A NEBULIZER

1   Wash your hands with soap and water.
2   Place the nebulizer on a hard surface, and make sure the air filter is clean.
3   Open the medication vial, and place the solution into the nebulizer container (called a cup).
4   Make sure the medication cup is connected to the nebulizer.
5   Place the mouthpiece into your mouth, and close your lips.
6   Turn on the nebulizer.
7   Breathe in and out normally.
8   Continue until the solution is gone (the nebulizer may begin to "sputter").
9   After each use, clean the medication cup with mild soap and water and allow to air dry.
10   Follow any other directions by the manufacturer for cleaning the nebulizer system.

Comparison of a pMDI and Nebulizer

Some individuals with asthma and COPD report that nebulized medications are more helpful in improving breathing difficulty compared with other delivery systems. It is important to recognize

Table 6.1 Comparison of doses of quick-acting bronchodilators by delivery system

	pMDI	NEBULIZER	DIFFERENCE
albuterol sulfate	2 puffs (180 µgm)	2,500 µgm	13.9 times
ipratropium bromide	2 puffs (36 µgm)	5,000 µgm	138.9 times

that the dose of the liquid medication used in a nebulizer is considerably higher than the dose of the same medication available in a pMDI. Two examples are shown in table 6.1.

As a result of the considerably higher doses, you may experience greater benefits but also more side effects with the same medication in a nebulizer than with the standard dose of two puffs of a pMDI. For a beta-agonist bronchodilator such as albuterol, you may experience shakiness and a rapid heart rate. For a muscarinic antagonist such as ipratropium, you may experience dryness of the mouth and difficulty with urination. You should discuss any concerns or questions with your health-care provider.

Key Points

> Different delivery systems of inhaler medications require different breathing techniques, as shown in table 6.2.

Table 6.2 Recommended inhalation techniques

DELIVERY SYSTEM	INHALATION TECHNIQUE
Pressurized metered-dose inhaler	slow and steady
Pressurized metered-dose inhaler with spacer	slow and steady
Respimat inhaler	slow and steady
Dry-powder inhaler	hard and fast
Solution in nebulizer	normal breathing in and out

> With a pMDI (with or without a spacer), Respimat inhaler, and DPI, you should hold your breath as long as possible. With a nebulizer, you breathe normally and there is no need to hold your breath.
> If you have questions or are uncertain if you are using the inhaler correctly, you should ask your health-care provider or nurse to watch you using the device.
> If the medication does not help you breathe easier, tell your health-care provider. One possibility is that you are not using the inhaler correctly.

References

Levy, Mark L., et al. "Inhaler Technique: Facts and Fantasies: A View from the Aerosol Drug Management Improvement Team (ADMIT)." *Primary Care Respiratory Medicine*, April 21, 2016. doi:10.1038 /npjpcrm.2016.17 (Epub ahead of print).

Melani, Andrea S., et al. "Inhaler Mishandling Remains Common in Real Life and Is Associated with Reduced Disease Control." *Respiratory Medicine* 106 (2012): 668–76.

Sanchis, Joaquin, Ignasi Gich, and Soren Pedersen. "Systematic Review of Errors in Inhaler Use: Has Patient Technique Improved Over Time?" *Chest* 150 (2016): 394–406.

Sims, Michael W. "Aerosol Therapy for Obstructive Lung Disease: Device Selection and Practice Management Issues." *Chest* 140 (2011): 781–88.

(7)

Interstitial Lung Disease

In the end it's not about how many breaths you took.
In the end it's about the moments that took your breath away.
folk wisdom

Interstitial lung disease is the name for a group of diseases that inflame or scar the lungs. The word *interstitial* refers to a lace-like network of tissue that supports the walls of the air sacs of the lungs (see figure 7.1). This is different than diseases such as asthma (chapter 4) or chronic obstructive pulmonary disease (COPD; chapter 5) that involve the breathing tubes (airways).

Inflammation (in Latin it means "set afire") is an important part of the body's immune system to heal an injury or fight an infection. It is essential to remove whatever caused the injury to the lung. As an example, inhaling fungal spores from moldy hay is one cause of interstitial lung disease. It is commonly called "farmer's lung." In an attempt to clear away the fungal spores, the body calls in (recruits) white blood cells to the area of the lung injury. This results in redness and swelling of the area—the features of inflammation. However, if inflammation persists and become chronic, it can damage the lung. Over time, inflammation can lead to scarring, a natural part of the body's repair process. Scarring in the lungs is called *pulmonary fibrosis.*

Both inflammation and scarring restrict the lung from expanding when you breathe in and make it hard to get enough oxygen into the blood. It is important for your health-care provider to try to distinguish whether there is mainly inflammation in the lungs or mainly scarring. *Why?* Inflammation can clear on its own with

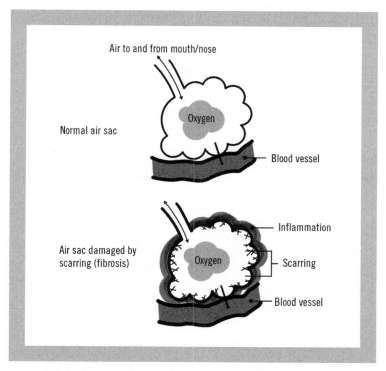

Figure 7.1 On the top is a normal air sac next to a blood vessel (pulmonary capillary). On the bottom is an air sac damaged by inflammation and scarring (cross-hatched areas) as occurs in interstitial lung disease. (LeftRightCreative)

time or with anti-inflammatory medications, such as prednisone. In contrast, scarring is permanent and cannot be reversed.

Causes

There are over two hundred different causes of interstitial lung disease. The major types are listed in table 7.1. Inhaling various materials as part of work or from the environment may trigger

Table 7.1 Major causes of interstitial lung disease

Occupational and environmental
> Asbestos fibers: from working with insulation and brake linings
> Coal dust: from working in a coal mine
> Grain dust: from farming
> Hypersensitivity pneumonitis: from inhaling dust, mold, or other irritants (common examples: droppings of pet birds and fungal spores from moldy hay)
> Silica fibers: from working in a granite mine
> Talc fibers: from working in a talc mine

Medications and radiation
> Antibiotics: one example is nitrofurantoin
> Anti-inflammatory: one example is sulfasalazine
> Chemotherapy drugs: methotrexate and cyclophosphamide are examples
> Heart medications: amiodarone

Autoimmune conditions
> Dermatomyositis and polymyositis
> Mixed-connective-tissue disease
> Pulmonary vasculitis
> Rheumatoid arthritis
> Sarcoidosis
> Scleroderma
> Sjogren's syndrome
> Systemic lupus erythematosus

Idiopathic interstitial pneumonias
> Acute interstitial pneumonitis
> Cryptogenic organizing pneumonitis
> Desquamative interstitial pneumonitis
> Idiopathic pulmonary fibrosis
> Nonspecific interstitial pneumonitis

Cancer
> Adenocarcinoma in situ
> Spread of cancer cells to the lymph channels (lymphatics) in the lungs

Other
> Lymphangioleiomyomatosis
> Neurofibromatosis
> Pulmonary alveolar proteinosis

an injury to the lungs that can lead to inflammation and possible scarring. For example, long-term inhalation of asbestos fibers, coal dust, silica fibers, and talc fibers can injure the lungs. Various medications may also cause interstitial lung disease. It is important to tell your health-care provider about all prescription and over-the-counter medications that you have taken or are currently using. Many of the connective-tissue diseases, such as rheumatoid arthritis and systemic lupus erythematosus, may also involve the lungs in addition to other parts of the body. Another category for interstitial lung disease is called idiopathic. The word *idiopathic* means that the cause is unknown. There are other less common causes that are not listed in table 7.1

Risk Factors

There are several risk factors that make it more likely for you to develop interstitial lung disease.

Age: more common in adults
Exposure to dusts, fibers, and fumes in the environment and
   with certain occupations
Family history: some forms of interstitial lung disease may be
   hereditary
Radiation treatments to the chest: as treatment for cancer
Cigarette smoking: some forms of interstitial lung disease are
   more likely in those who smoke or have smoked

Symptoms

The two main symptoms of interstitial lung disease are a cough and shortness of breath. The cough is usually "dry." Many people wait to tell their health-care provider about their shortness of breath until it interferes with daily activities. Make sure to mention any cough that persists as well as any breathing difficulty.

Your health-care provider may suspect interstitial lung disease if he or she hears "crackling" sounds when listening to your chest with a stethoscope. A chest x-ray typically shows increased lines or shadows in the lungs. Your health-care provider may ask questions, such as those listed here, in order to try to figure out a possible cause for your interstitial lung disease.

When did your symptoms start?

What medications and supplements are you taking? What medications have you taken in the past, including over-the-counter medications?

What is your occupation? What type of work did you do in the past?

Do you use a hot tub? Do you use an air conditioner or humidifier?

Do you have pet birds?

Do any of your family members have a lung disease?

Have you ever received radiation treatments or chemotherapy?

Do you have other medical conditions?

Testing

Your oxygen saturation can be measured by an oximeter placed on the finger at rest and when walking (see chapter 3). In healthy individuals, the oxygen saturation remains the same at rest and with walking. In those with interstitial lung disease, the oxygen level usually falls with activities. This measurement can also determine whether you should use oxygen at rest or with activities. Certain breathing tests are important to determine whether the lungs are restricted from full expansion (called lung volumes) and whether carbon monoxide (as a substitute gas for oxygen) is impaired when moving from the air sacs into the blood vessels of the lungs (called diffusing capacity).

Identifying the exact cause of interstitial lung disease can be challenging. Blood tests can be useful in certain diseases such as exposure to bird protein or moldy hay, sarcoidosis, connective tissue diseases, and vasculitis. A chest x-ray may show characteristic changes, but a high-resolution computerized tomography (CT) scan of the chest can provide detailed information about location and extent of the interstitial disease that can help to determine a specific cause. Your primary care provider may refer you to a lung specialist (pulmonologist) for evaluation.

Depending on the results of these tests, your health-care provider or the lung specialist may recommend a biopsy of the lungs to find out a specific cause. The biopsy obtains one or more pieces of lung tissue to look at under the microscope. This is done by either passing a scope through the mouth into the lungs (called bronchoscopy) or an operation (called thorascopy). With thorascopy, the surgeon places medical instruments and a camera through small incisions between ribs to remove tissue samples from the lung.

Idiopathic Pulmonary Fibrosis

Idiopathic pulmonary fibrosis is a specific type of interstitial lung disease. As mentioned earlier in the chapter, *idiopathic* means that the cause is unknown. Pulmonary fibrosis means there is scarring of the lung. A CT scan of the chest in someone with idiopathic pulmonary fibrosis is shown in figure 7.2. The condition typically occurs in people over the age of fifty and tends to affect slightly more men than women. It is believed that this condition starts with an injury to the lining of the air sacs (alveoli). Although the body attempts to heal the injury, the repair leads to scarring. The reason that scarring occurs is not well understood.

Figure 7.2 View of a CT scan of the chest in someone with idiopathic pulmonary fibrosis. There are increased linear markings in both lungs and small cysts toward the bottom of the lungs. This is called honeycombing. (Wikimedia Commons /IPFeditor)

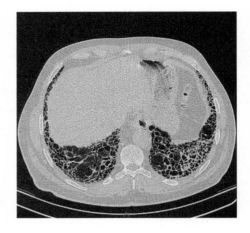

A Possible Cause for Idiopathic Pulmonary Fibrosis: Gastroesophageal Reflux

One possible consideration for idiopathic pulmonary fibrosis is aspiration of acid into the lungs. *How does this happen?* Acid is normally produced in the stomach to help digest food. Acid in the stomach can reflux back into the swallowing tube (esophagus) as shown in figure 7.3. This is called gastroesophageal reflux disease (abbreviated GERD). The usual symptoms of acid moving up into the swallowing tube (esophagus) are heartburn and indigestion. However, some individuals with idiopathic pulmonary fibrosis may have "silent" reflux and do not have any symptoms. In some cases, the acid may reflux into the swallowing tube, move all the way up into the throat, and then slip down into the lungs. This process is called aspiration.

Acid is irritating and can cause injury to the air sacs of the lungs, especially if the person is susceptible to developing pulmonary fibrosis. Recurrent aspiration can be a repeated "trigger" for lung injury.

The main test to diagnose acid reflux is to place a small sensor

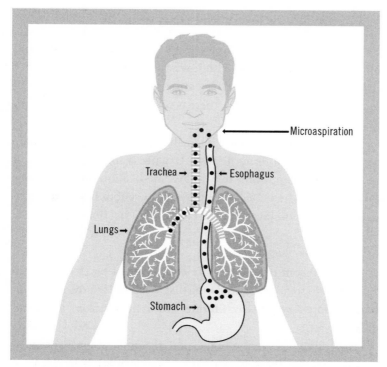

Figure 7.3 Connection between the stomach, swallowing tube (esophagus), and the respiratory tract. Acid in the stomach can reflux into the esophagus and may then slip into the windpipe (trachea) and down into the lungs. (Based on iStock.com images from elenabs and kowalska-art)

in the lower swallowing tube (esophagus) to monitor for acid reflux. This test is called esophageal pH monitoring. It is typically performed or supervised by a specialist (gastroenterologist). If there is evidence of acid reflux, there are both medical and surgical treatments.

The course of idiopathic pulmonary fibrosis varies from one person to another. However, it usually gets worse (progressive), causing more coughing and shortness of breath. On average, survival is about three years once the diagnosis is made.

Treatments for Interstitial Lung Disease

The following information provides an overall approach and options for treating those with interstitial lung disease. Some of these medications are used in an attempt to reduce inflammation in the lung. As stated earlier, there is no treatment to reverse scarring in the lungs.

Certain medications have been shown to be useful in specific types of interstitial lung disease. Usually, a lung specialist will recommend therapy and may adjust medication based on your response. You should ask the lung specialist about expected benefits as well as possible side effects of any medications prescribed.

MEDICATIONS

At the present time, there are two different types of medications used to treat interstitial lung disease: anti-inflammatory/immunosuppressive and antifibrotic. These medications are listed in table 7.2.

Corticosteroids are the major oral anti-inflammatory medication used when there is evidence of inflammation in the lung or if inflammation is suspected based on test results. In some causes (e.g., cryptogenic organizing pneumonitis, hypersensitivity pneumonitis, and sarcoidosis), prednisone can have a prompt and dramatic benefit in improving symptoms and clearing up the inflammation in the lungs. Other anti-inflammatory or immunosuppressive medications may be used for specific types of interstitial lung disease or because of concerns of side effects of prednisone. For example, cyclophosphamide and mycophenolate mofetil have been used to treat those with interstitial lung disease associated with scleroderma. Rituximab has been used in those with interstitial lung disease who do not respond to standard immunosuppressive medications listed in table 7.2.

Table 7.2 Medications used to treat interstitial lung disease

GENERIC NAME	BRAND NAME
Anti-inflammatory/immunosuppressive	
Azathioprine	Imuran
Corticosteroids	Prednisone
Cyclophosphamide	Cytoxan
Methotrexate	Otrexup; Rasuvo
Mycophenolate mofetil	Cellcept; Myfortic
Antifibrotic	
Nintedanib	Ofev
Pirfenidone	Esbriet

Prednisone is not recommended to treat those with idiopathic pulmonary fibrosis because there is no inflammation in this condition. Two medications—nintedanib and pirfenidone—have been approved as antifibrotic medications. This means that these medications will slow the development of scarring in the lungs but will not improve shortness of breath or the ability to do daily activities. Nintedanib is taken by mouth twice a day, while pirfenidone is taken by mouth three times a day. Each medication may cause possible side effects. You should ask your health-care provider about any possible problems while taking these medications.

OXYGEN

The need for oxygen in those with interstitial lung disease is assessed in the same manner as for other lung conditions. In general, an oxygen saturation of 88 percent or lower qualifies someone to use oxygen therapy. Many individuals who are diagnosed with interstitial lung disease have adequate levels of oxygen saturation at rest (89 percent or higher), but their saturation level falls with activities such as walking and possibly during sleep. Your health-care provider can evaluate your need for oxygen therapy and prescribe oxygen for you based on results.

LUNG TRANSPLANTATION

Those with advanced interstitial lung disease and no other major medical problems are candidates for lung transplantation. Idiopathic pulmonary fibrosis is the most common type of interstitial lung disease for which lung transplantation is considered. In general, candidates are short of breath during activities of daily living, are getting worse despite available treatment, and have a life expectancy of less than two years.

Each transplant center has slightly different criteria for who qualifies. Some centers will perform lung transplantation in those in their seventies if the individual is otherwise in good health. Usually, one lung is transplanted in those with idiopathic pulmonary fibrosis.

Complications

Interstitial lung disease can lead to some serious complications. These include a sudden worsening (exacerbation), high blood pressure in blood vessels of the lungs (pulmonary hypertension), and respiratory failure.

EXACERBATION

A sudden worsening can occur quite unexpectedly in many types of interstitial lung disease. Typically, the individual becomes more short of breath, and a chest x-ray or CT scan shows more lines or shadows without evidence of pneumonia, blood clots (pulmonary embolism), or heart failure. This happens in 5–15 percent of those with idiopathic pulmonary fibrosis each year. If the exacerbation is severe, it may require hospitalization with supportive care.

PULMONARY HYPERTENSION

This typically occurs if scar tissue or low oxygen levels restrict blood flow through the small blood vessels (pulmonary capillaries). This raises the pressure within the pulmonary arteries and puts a strain on the right side of the heart. If the pressure is high enough over a long time period, the right ventricle may enlarge and even fail. This can lead to swelling of the feet and legs. Medications that open narrowed blood vessels in the lung (called vasodilators) may provide some short-term benefit.

RESPIRATORY FAILURE

Respiratory failure means that the lungs are unable to maintain an adequate level of oxygen in the body or are unable to eliminate enough carbon dioxide. If this happens, the individual will experience more breathing difficulty. If respiratory failure occurs, then the individual and family members should discuss treatment options with the health-care provider or whether death appears to be likely. A decision is then needed regarding use of life support (such as a breathing machine) or whether palliative care and comfort measures should be provided.

Key Points

> Interstitial refers to a lacelike network of tissue that supports the air sacs (alveoli) in the lungs.
> Interstitial lung disease is a result of an injury that occurs in the air sacs (alveoli) that leads to inflammation or scarring (fibrosis).
> There are over two hundred different causes of interstitial lung disease.
> Both inflammation and scarring restrict the lung from expanding when someone breathes in. It also makes it hard to get enough oxygen into the blood.

> The main symptoms are a dry cough and shortness of breath with activities.
> Idiopathic pulmonary fibrosis is the most common type of interstitial lung disease.
> The cause of idiopathic pulmonary fibrosis is unknown, and there is no cure.
> Anti-inflammatory/immunosuppressive medications are used to treat those with interstitial lung disease who have inflammation or if inflammation is suspected.
> Antifibrotic medications are used to slow down worsening (progression) in those with idiopathic pulmonary fibrosis.
> Other treatments for interstitial lung disease include oxygen, pulmonary rehabilitation, and lung transplantation.
> Complications of interstitial lung disease are sudden worsening (exacerbation), high pressure in the blood vessels of the lungs (pulmonary hypertension), and respiratory failure.

References

Ghebre, Yohannes T., and Ganesh Raghu. "Idiopathic Pulmonary Fibrosis: Novel Concepts of Proton Pump Inhibitors as Antifibrotic Drugs." *American Journal of Respiratory and Critical Care Medicine* 193 (2016): 1345–52.

Hoeper, Marius M. "Pulmonary Hypertension in Patients with Chronic Fibrosing Idiopathic Interstitial Pneumonias." *PLoS One* 10 (2015): e0141911.

Raghu, Ganesh, et al. "An Official ATS/ERS/JRS/ALAT Clinical Practice Guideline: Treatment of Idiopathic Pulmonary Fibrosis; An Update of the 2011 Clinical Practice Guideline." *American Journal of Respiratory and Critical Care Medicine* 192 (2015): e3–e19.

Ryerson, Christopher J., Vincent Cottin, Kevin K. Brown, and Harold R. Collard. "Acute Exacerbation of Idiopathic Pulmonary Fibrosis: Shifting the Paradigm." *European Respiratory Journal* 46 (2015): 512–20.

(8)

Will Exercise Help?

Exercise is the single best thing you can do for your brain in terms of mood, memory, and learning.

Dr. John Ratey, psychiatrist and author (1948–)

If I knew I was going to live this long, I'd have taken better care of myself.

Mickey Mantle, baseball player for New York Yankees (1931–1995)

Everyone knows about exercise. As kids, it is called playing. Almost all children love to play outside, both organized sports and games. "Hide and seek" and "kick the can" are old-time favorites. These activities involve running, jumping, and having a strategy to beat siblings and neighbors. Riding bikes in the neighborhood was a ritual of summer for many.

Then what happens? People reach adulthood and are busy with work, relationships, and family. Some adults continue to play games such as soccer, basketball, or tennis, while others enjoy running or biking. Many go to fitness centers to work out on their own or join exercise classes. However, a majority avoids any and all unnecessary physical activities for a variety of reasons.

The demands of work and family frequently "get in the way" and limit both time and energy so that playing pick-up games or exercising regularly becomes a major challenge.

For health and fitness, the American College of Sports Medicine offers guidance for exercise in healthy adults. The statement concludes that "the scientific evidence demonstrating the beneficial effects of exercise is indisputable, and the benefits far

outweigh the risks in most adults." The following recommendations also apply to adults with chronic diseases.

The American College of Sports Medicine recommends that
adults engage in

moderate-intensity exercise for at least thirty minutes per day for
   at least five days per week (total of 150 minutes per week);
   OR
vigorous intensity exercise for at least twenty minutes per day for
   at least three days per week (total of seventy-five minutes per
   week);
   OR
a combination of moderate and vigorous exercise to achieve
   a total energy expenditure of five hundred to one thousand
   metabolic equivalents (MET) per week.

In addition to the above exercise options, resistance (strength)
training is recommended for each of the major muscle groups two
to three days per week. The statement goes on to comment that
adults who are unable or unwilling to meet the exercise targets
listed above can still benefit from engaging in amounts of exercise
less than what is recommended.

According to the Centers for Disease Control (CDC), the majority of adults in the United States do not meet recommended exercise targets. In general, the percentages of adults who achieve the
exercise recommendations decline with age. In the report from
the CDC, only 16 percent of adults between the ages of fifty-five
and seventy-four participated in 150 minutes of aerobic exercise
per week.

Certainly, if you have a respiratory illness such as asthma,
COPD, or interstitial lung disease, you know that various physical
activities will cause you to feel short of breath. The natural tendency is to then avoid activities (e.g., climbing the stairs, carrying
packages, housework, or yard work) that bring on this unpleas-

ant experience. Unfortunately, the less you do, the less you are able to do.

Deconditioning describes the decline in the body's ability to perform physical tasks that occurs with inactivity. This might occur by choice ("I don't have enough time" or "I don't feel like it") or result from injury or illness. For example, a "chest cold" causes not only breathing difficulty, coughing, and chest pain but also fatigue and low energy that can linger for weeks. As a result, the inactivity may be enough to cause muscle weakness, poor energy, and a feeling of tiredness. For example, you lose 10–20 percent of your muscle strength each week that you are inactive. The different levels of deconditioning are as follows:

Mild: difficulty with exercise
Moderate: difficulty with normal activities (e.g., walking,
    shopping, yard work, and housework)
Severe: difficulty with minimal activities and self-care

This chapter reviews the effects of aging on the brain and the body. An understanding of what happens as you get older provides a background for appreciating the multiple benefits of regular exercise. Specific information is provided about the reasons that everyone with a chronic lung condition should participate in pulmonary rehabilitation. Suggestions are made about how to continue exercise if you decide that it is easier or more convenient to do this on your own rather than participate in a pulmonary rehabilitation program. For many individuals, there are advantages if the exercise program is supervised by a health professional or fitness specialist who can provide information, support, and encouragement. There are also many social benefits of group activities.

Effects of Aging

The effects of aging on the brain and the body are well defined. The major changes are listed in table 8.1. However, it is important to remember that what happens in real life is usually a combination of getting older along with reduced physical activity. Moreover, the changes described in table 8.1 are quite variable among individuals because of genetics, lifestyle, and diet.

By observing your parents, any older siblings, relatives, and those living in the community, you have a glimpse of the future and what might, or could, happen as you get older. Some of these changes may be obvious, while others are quite subtle.

THE BRAIN

The changes that occur in the brain with aging influence learning, memory, planning, and other mental activities. For example, it might take longer to learn or remember new information, and

Table 8.1 General changes with aging

INCREASES	DECREASES
In the Brain	
Plaques develop outside of neurons	Size of the brain (prefrontal cortex and hippocampus)
Inflammation	Memory
	Learning new tasks
	Blood flow because arteries narrow
	Reflexes slow
In the Body	
Body weight	Body height
Percent body fat	Muscle strength and flexibility
Stiffness of blood vessels	Lung function

you might have difficulty remembering familiar words or names of people.

Fortunately, certain brain regions can become active in older adults to compensate for difficulties in other areas of the brain. For example, the brain may recruit different networks of brain cells in order to perform a task. This is called *neuroplasticity*. In simple terms, the brain is like muscle in your body, "Use it or lose it."

THE BODY

As you get older, total body weight, which reflects the number of calories that you eat and the number of calories that you use or burn, generally increases. Without exercise, added weight is stored as fat rather than muscle. Body fat generally shifts to the midsection or belly (figure 8.1).

This is often referred to as an "apple" shape. "Belly fat" includes fat under the skin as well as what accumulates around the internal organs (for example, the liver and intestines) within the abdomen.

Why is this important? If most of your fat is around your waist rather than at your hips, you're at a higher risk for heart disease

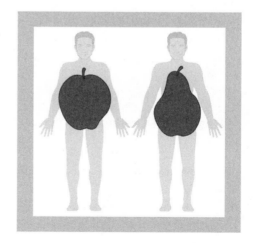

Figure 8.1 General types of extra body fat described as "apple" and "pear" shapes. (Based on iStock.com images from elenabs, kowalska-art, and sssimone)

and type 2 diabetes. This risk goes up with a waist size that is greater than thirty-five inches for women or greater than forty inches for men. For example, among the forty-four thousand women in the Nurses' Health Study, those with greater waist size (waist circumference) were more likely to die of heart disease and cancer than women with smaller waists.

Muscle accounts for 40–50 percent of total body weight in a healthy adult. In general, there is a 1 percent loss of muscle mass each year after the age of thirty. Since muscle burns more calories than fat, this has implications for overall weight. In addition, muscles lose strength and flexibility with aging. Coordination and balance may also be affected.

You also get shorter as you age. In general, you lose half an inch every ten years after the age of forty. This means that you may lose one to three inches of height over a lifetime. This is because the discs between the vertebrae in the spine dehydrate and shrink. The aging spine can also become more curved, and vertebrae can collapse due to loss of bone density.

Lung function (measured by breathing tests) declines slowly after fifty years of age. Because blood vessels become stiffer as you get older, the heart has to work harder to pump blood through them. This can lead to high blood pressure (hypertension). Constipation is common in older adults. Bladder function can change with aging as women are affected by menopause and men by an enlarged prostate gland.

Benefits of Exercise

There are numerous benefits of regular exercise for both the mind and the body. Exercise can increase your energy level, improve your outlook, and help you lose weight. It has been called the *fountain of youth*. The benefits of exercise on the mind are truly remarkable:

Makes you happier and smarter
Keeps the brain fit
Improves learning
Lifts depression
Reverses stress
Improves self-esteem and body image

Harvard Medical School psychiatrist Dr. John Ratey said, "Exercise is the single best thing you can do for your brain in terms of mood, memory, and learning." *Why?* Exercise increases blood flow to the brain and also increases levels of certain chemicals, called growth factors, which help to make new brain cells and new connections (networks) between brain cells. According to Ratey, "Like muscles, you have to stress your brain cells to get them to grow."

How does exercise affect the mind? Research shows that burning 350 calories three times a week through sustained activity that makes you sweat can reduce symptoms of depression about as effectively as antidepressant medications. Exercise appears to stimulate the growth of neurons in certain brain regions affected by depression. Three sessions of yoga per week has been shown to boost levels of the brain chemical GABA, which typically translates into improved mood and decreased anxiety. In addition, exercise can increase levels of "feel-good" chemicals such as serotonin, dopamine, and beta-endorphins.

The benefits of exercise on the body are numerous and impressive. Some people might spend a lot of money if a daily pill was available to achieve just a few of these positive effects:

1 Prevents heart disease and stroke by
   > lowering blood pressure,
   > raising high-density lipoprotein (HDL)—"good cholesterol"
   > lowering low-density lipoprotein (LDL)—"bad cholesterol"
   > increasing the working capacity of the heart
2 Prevents and controls diabetes mellitus

3 Controls weight and reduces body fat
4 Improves the body's ability to burn calories
5 Weight-bearing exercise promotes bone strength and prevents fractures.
6 Reduces the risk of colon cancer, breast cancer, uterine cancer, and lung cancer
7 Promotes better sleep
8 Improves sexual interest

How does exercise reduce the risk of cancer? There is no proven way to completely prevent cancer, but exercise can help lower your risk. This occurs by preventing obesity, reducing inflammation and hormone levels in the body, improving insulin resistance, and improving immune function. For colon cancer, people who exercise regularly have a 40–50 percent lower risk of this cancer compared to those who don't exercise regularly. For breast cancer, moderate to vigorous exercise for more than three hours per week provides a 30–40 percent lower risk. There is a 38–46 percent reduced risk of uterine cancer in active women. Studies show that people who are regularly active are less likely to develop lung cancer, which may be related to being less likely to smoke and use tobacco products.

Pulmonary Rehabilitation

If you have a chronic respiratory condition, such as asthma, COPD, or interstitial lung disease, and are affected by shortness of breath with activities, it may be difficult to imagine starting an exercise program. A typical comment is, "If I have a problem breathing during daily activities, how can I even consider exercise?" The answer to that question is that starting an exercise program is an investment in your health. You can expect some improvements in just a few weeks, and there are many long-term health benefits as described earlier in this chapter.

The best way to get started is to join a pulmonary rehabilitation program. Health insurance companies typically pay for participation in pulmonary rehabilitation. These programs are usually available at hospitals and medical centers. The goal is to "restore the person to the highest possible level of independent function." This is accomplished by helping individuals become physically active and to learn more about their disease, treatments, and how to cope. Anyone with a stable chronic lung disease who is affected by shortness of breath should consider participating in pulmonary rehabilitation.

A successful program has three major components:

multidisciplinary: includes expertise from various health-care
    disciplines including nursing, respiratory care, physical
    therapy, occupational therapy, nutrition, and exercise science;
individualized: each person's needs and goals are assessed, and
    an exercise program is designed to help you achieve realistic
    goals; and
a focus on physical and social function: includes attention to
    physical impairment as well as psychological, emotional, and
    social problems.

The established benefits of participation in pulmonary rehabilitation are as follows:

Reduces breathlessness
Improves quality of life
Increases exercise capacity
Reduces the risk of a COPD exacerbation
Increases muscle strength
Improves psychosocial function

Being able to do more with less breathing difficulty is very important. Strengthening the leg and arm muscles with training results in increased exercise capacity even though there is no change in how your lungs work. The improved efficiency of these muscles leads to a reduced level of breathing required to perform a physical task. For example, before pulmonary rehabilitation you may need to breathe fifteen liters each minute while walking on the level; after an eight-week program, you may only require to breathe ten to twelve liters each minute. This means that there is less demand on your respiratory system and that it will be easier to breathe with activities.

Components of Pulmonary Rehabilitation

Exercise training is considered the cornerstone of a pulmonary rehabilitation program. Typically, exercise includes leg activities such as walking on a treadmill, pedaling a stationary cycle, and using a step or elliptical machine. In addition, many activities of daily living involve use of the arms. For this reason, programs include upper-extremity exercises such as lifting weights, use of elastic bands, and arm-crank machines. As you know, exercise only benefits the actual muscles doing the work. This is called *specificity* of training.

The American Thoracic and the European Respiratory Societies have provided recommendations for frequency, intensity, and duration of exercise training as part of pulmonary rehabilitation. These guidelines are listed in table 8.2. The specific recommendations are similar for intensity and duration of exercise training as published by the American College of Sports Medicine (see above) for healthy adults. However, the recommended number of exercise sessions per week is less (should be at least three times per week). Certainly, exercising more frequently provides greater benefits.

Your pulmonary rehabilitation coordinator may modify the specific recommendations based on your abilities and motivation. It is important to remember that *getting started* is key. You

Table 8.2 Recommendations for pulmonary rehabilitation

Aerobic Exercise

Frequency: at least three times each week (although more is better)

Intensity: at least 60 percent of peak exercise capacity OR level of breathlessness (rating of 4–6) on the 0–10 scale by Borg

Duration: 20–60 minutes of exercise per session

Interval Training (an alternative to aerobic exercise)

Several 30–60-second bouts of high-intensity exercise with periods of rest or lower exercise intensity between efforts

Strength Training

Two to four sets of six to twelve repetitions of major muscle groups at each training session

Involves both weights and stretch bands. This is usually done after aerobic exercise training.

---

can work toward achieving the recommendations over time. Ideally, you should attend at least three exercise sessions per week that are supervised by a health professional. However, two supervised sessions per week is considered acceptable along with one or more sessions on your own at home or at a fitness center. Sessions typically include warm-up, exercise training, cooldown, stretching, strength training, and education about different aspects of respiratory disease. These sessions usually last one and a half to two hours. In general, for exercise training, "more is better." As examples, twenty sessions have been shown to provide greater improvements than ten sessions, and higher-intensity training produces greater physiological benefits than lower-intensity exertion.

The intensity of training (how hard you are working) is a key consideration of exercise. It is reasonable for most individuals to start with low-intensity training, especially if you have not been physically active and are not used to "pushing yourself." The low-intensity approach allows you to improve slowly and gain confidence without being exhausted after each session. The pulmonary rehabilitation program director will discuss the exercise intensity with you at the first session and will monitor you by checking your heart rate, blood pressure, and oxygen saturation, and asking you to rate your breathing difficulty during exercise.

Two basic approaches are used for you to monitor how hard to exercise. One is to rate your breathing difficulty on a scale (such as the zero-to-ten scale developed by Professor Gunnar Borg of Sweden) while you exercise. Usually the program coordinator will hold the scale in front of you so that you can report your breathing difficulty every few minutes or so. The goal is to work at a tolerable level of breathlessness in order to improve. Although the recommended rating of breathlessness is four to six on the Borg scale (see table 8.2), I consider this intensity to be higher than can be tolerated for twenty to sixty minutes of exercise for many individuals. In general, it is hard for someone to sustain "severe" breathlessness (a rating of five) for the target of at least twenty minutes of exertion. Instead, I suggest that a level of three, or "moderate" breathlessness on the Borg scale, is more appropriate and realistic when you start a rehabilitation program.

An alternative approach is to use your heart rate at a guide. This requires a heart-rate monitor (chest strap or wristband) or oximeter (measures heart rate as well as oxygen saturation). The target heart rate for training can be selected as the measured heart rate at a percentage (typically at least 60 percent) of maximal exercise capacity during a cardiopulmonary exercise test. The program coordinator will tell you what the target heart rate is for you. He or she should discuss these different approaches with you and provide guidance during your exercise sessions.

If you are using long-term oxygen therapy, then oxygen should be continued during the exercise sessions. It is likely that you will need to increase the flow rate that you use at rest while you exercise in order to keep the saturation at or above 90 percent. If you are not currently using oxygen, but your oxygen saturation drops to 88 percent or below during exercise, then oxygen will be prescribed during training sessions. The goal is to keep the oxygen saturation close to 92 percent or above while you exercise in order to make it easier to breathe and to allow you to do more work.

The minimal goal for duration is at least twenty minutes of exertion. How long you can exercise depends on how hard it is (the intensity). The twenty-minute target may be nonstop (continuous) doing one activity, or it may be a combination of activities, such as walking on the treadmill for ten minutes and then pedaling on a stationary cycle for ten more minutes. For some individuals, especially at the initial visits, twenty minutes of exercise may not be possible. Rather, it may be reasonable to do ten to twenty minutes of combined exercise with rest periods at the first several visits, while you build endurance and stamina. It may also take several weeks for you to achieve the twenty-minutes target. This often depends on how fit or how active you are at the start of pulmonary rehabilitation. Hopefully, you will be able to exercise longer each week as you become familiar with the equipment, are more comfortable and relaxed, and gain confidence.

Strength training is an important part of pulmonary rehabilitation. Training sessions usually include two to four sets with each set being six to twelve repetitions. Figure 8.2 shows people using dumbbells for arm exercises. The program director will help you select the weight of the dumbbell at the beginning of pulmonary rehabilitation. It is important to remember that strong muscles are able to perform a physical task easier and can function for longer periods of time without getting tired. Good muscle strength also enhances posture and may help to prevent injuries.

The following points summarize important information about your participation in pulmonary rehabilitation.

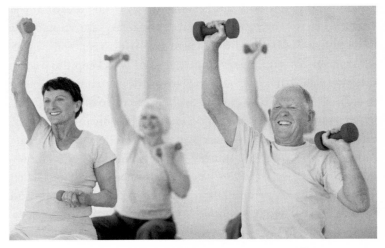

Figure 8.2 Group exercise using weights to improve strength
(iStock.com/kupicoo)

At the first or screening visit, the program director will ask,
"What are your goals?" You should think about what specific
activities are most important to your daily life. Your desire to
improve should be motivation for pushing yourself on those
days when you might feel tired.

A minimum of twenty supervised sessions is recommended to
achieve benefits. This can be three times per week, or two
supervised sessions per week plus one unsupervised home
session.

High-intensity exercise leads to greater benefits. However,
low-intensity training is quite effective, and you will likely
be able to do it for a longer time.

Training should include both arms and legs.

Endurance and strength training lead to complementary
improvements in muscle function.

Hopefully, you will have fun participating with others who are
also working to improve.

Education is part of a pulmonary rehabilitation program that promotes adaptive behaviors such as self-efficacy. Self-efficacy is the confidence in being able to successfully manage your health. Certainly, the more you know about your condition, the better you are able to participate with your health-care provider to manage the illness and any complications. Self-management includes problem solving, decision making, and taking action according to a specific plan. This typically includes what to do if your breathing gets worse, what to do if you cough up yellow or green mucus, and when to call your health-care provider for advice and help. This is generally called an action plan.

After You Complete Pulmonary Rehabilitation

It is important to continue exercise training after you finish pulmonary rehabilitation. If you stop exercising after you complete the program, you will gradually lose whatever you gained. The benefits of pulmonary rehabilitation decline over six to twelve months if you do not continue with exercise. Ideally, you should consider pulmonary rehabilitation to be a start of a lifelong choice to maintain a healthy lifestyle. Some pulmonary rehabilitation programs allow individuals to continue to use the facility and equipment as part of maintenance phase. Typically, the sessions are less supervised and may require a minimal fee.

If you decide to exercise on your own, one challenge is to know how hard to push yourself. If it too easy, there is little or no benefit. If it too hard, it is difficult to sustain over weeks to months. You should use the same approach—ratings of breathlessness or heart rate—that you used during participation in pulmonary rehabilitation. Both approaches depend on monitoring the responses of your body. Monitoring your breathing difficulty requires attention to how bad and how unpleasant your breathing feels during exercise.

Key Points

> Aging affects both the brain and the body. However, the aging process is quite variable among individuals.

> *Deconditioning* refers to the loss of fitness that occurs with inactivity. It is common in adults and may occur by choice ("I don't have enough time") or result from an injury or illness.

> For health and basic fitness, the American College of Sports Medicine has recommended at least thirty minutes of *moderate*-intensity aerobic exercise at least five days per week (total of 150 minutes per week), or at least thirty minutes of *vigorous*-intensity exercise at least three days per week (total of ninety minutes per week).

> Regular exercise benefits both the brain and the body. Exercise can help people lose weight, increase energy, and improve outlook. It has been called the *fountain of youth*.

> Anyone with a chronic respiratory illness should consider participating in a pulmonary rehabilitation program.

> Pulmonary rehabilitation is multidisciplinary, is individualized, and attends to psychological, emotional, and social issues. It includes aerobic exercise, strength training, and education.

> Recommendations for pulmonary rehabilitation include at least three sessions a week; exercise at 60 percent of your peak exercise capacity; at least twenty minutes per session; and strength training at each session.

References

Garber, Carol Ewing, et al. "Quantity and Quality of Exercise for Developing and Maintaining Cardiorespiratory, Musculoskeletal, and Neuromotor Fitness in Apparently Healthy Adults: Guidance for Prescribing Exercise." *Medicine and Science in Sports and Exercise* 43 (2011): 1334–59.

Grundy, Scott M., et al. "Diagnosis and Management of the Metabolic Syndrome: An American Heart Association/National Heart, Lung, and Blood Institute Scientific Statement." *Circulation* 112, no. 17 (2005): 2735–52.

Nici, Linda, et al. "American Thoracic Society/European Respiratory Society Statement on Pulmonary Rehabilitation." *American Journal of Respiratory and Critical Care Medicine* 173 (2006): 1390–1413.

Ratey, John J., and Eric Hageman. *SPARK: The Revolutionary New Science of Exercise and the Brain.* New York: Little, Brown, 2008.

Spruit, Martin A., et al. "An Official American Thoracic Society/European Respiratory Society Statement: Key Concepts and Advances in Pulmonary Rehabilitation." *American Journal of Respiratory and Critical Care Medicine* 188 (2013): 1011–27.

Wadell, Karin, Katherine A. Webb, Megan E. Preston, and Denis E. O'Donnell. "Impact of Pulmonary Rehabilitation on the Major Dimensions of Dyspnea in COPD." *COPD* 10 (2013): 425–35.

Zhang, Cuilin, et al. "Abdominal Obesity and the Risk of All-Cause, Cardiovascular, and Cancer Mortality: Sixteen Years of Follow-up in US Women." *Circulation* 117, no. 13 (2008): 1658–67.

(9)

Other Strategies to Relieve Shortness of Breath

> Breath is the finest gift of nature. Be grateful to the
> supreme for this wonderful gift.
>
> Amit Ray, author of books on meditation (1960–)

This chapter describes a variety of strategies that you can try or consider to relieve your shortness of breath. For some of these treatments, there is good evidence of benefit for helping breathlessness. For others, the treatment might help, but studies are either lacking or show inconsistent results.

It is also important to understand that results from studies provide an overall effect based on the types of participants in the study. However, everyone is an individual, and a particular strategy or treatment may or may not work to relieve breathing difficulty. Often, a treatment needs to be tried to find out if it helps you breathe easier. If it does not, then it should be stopped and another strategy should be considered.

I have divided these "other strategies" for relief of shortness of breath into three categories:

simple and inexpensive,
treatments for those with specific conditions, and
emerging strategies.

The simple and inexpensive strategies should be tried first. Next, you should consider treatments depending on your individual situation. You will likely need to consult your health-care provider to find out if you qualify or fit any of these specific conditions. Emerging therapies offer potential or theoretical benefits, but the scientific evidence is lacking. As a result, you might consider emerging therapies based on your interest and available expertise in the area where you live.

Simple and Inexpensive Strategies

AIR MOVEMENT

Many individuals find that sitting in front of an open window with a breeze helps to make breathing easier. Similarly, having a fan blow air on the face reduces breathing discomfort. In one study, a handheld fan directed to the face reduced the reports of breathlessness in fifty subjects who had advanced heart or lung disease.

ACTIVITIES THAT PROMOTE
RELEASE OF ENDORPHINS

Endorphins are naturally occurring substances in the body that act like morphine. They are released into the brain in response to pain or stress. For example, endorphin levels increase in response to surgery, an injury like a bone fracture, and exercise. The release of endorphins that occurs with physical exercise is presumably the cause for the feeling of a "runner's high." A specific stress that also stimulates release of endorphins is breathing difficulty. Studies show that endorphins relieve the severity of breathlessness in those with chronic obstructive pulmonary disease (COPD).

Thus, the body produces endorphin substances in order to reduce unpleasant experiences such as pain and shortness of breath. In addition, endorphins are responsible, in part, for pleasure or "feeling good" when, for example, we eat certain foods. Various "triggers" that stimulate release of endorphins into the body include the following:

Acupuncture
Alcohol
Caffeine
Chili peppers containing capsaicin
Dark chocolate
Exercise
Laughter
Listening to soothing music
Massage
Meditation and controlled-breathing exercises (e.g., Tai Chi,
    Pilates, and yoga)
Ultraviolet light

Several studies show that acupuncture reduces breathlessness in those with COPD. This is discussed later in this chapter. Light to moderate drinking of alcohol produces a "buzz" that may be related to the release of endorphins in the brain.

Some people claim to be "addicted" to eating chocolate. In particular, dark chocolate has proven health benefits that are likely due to flavonoids. Flavonoids are antioxidants that help to protect the body from damage by free radicals. Dark chocolate contains more cocoa, and thus more flavonoids, than milk chocolate. Eating dark chocolate stimulates a release of endorphins, which then causes a release of serotonin. Both endorphins and serotonin improve mood and provide a pleasurable feeling.

It is interesting that exposure to ultraviolet light releases endorphins. This may be one reason some people lie in the sun or use a tanning bed regularly. However, ultraviolet light can cause premature aging to the skin and increase the risk of skin cancer.

Whether release of endorphins with these "triggers" reduces breathlessness is an interesting possibility. However, at the present time there is little, if any, evidence that these "triggers" help breathing difficulty except for acupuncture. You may wish to try

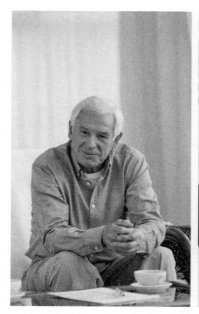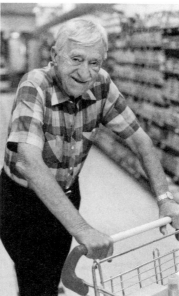

Figure 9.1 On the left is a man leaning forward with forearms supported on his thighs; this is called the tripod position. On the right, a man supports his hands on a shopping cart. These positions can make it easier to breathe. (Based on iStock.com images mediaphotos and RapidEye)

one or more of these activities and observe whether there is any change in your shortness of breath.

BODY POSITION

Leaning forward with hands or forearms resting on an object can provide some relief of breathlessness. One common position is for the arms to rest on the thighs. Many individuals find they can walk a longer distance with less breathlessness when their hands hold on to a shopping cart (figure 9.1). Studies suggest that postural relief of breathing difficulty may be related to improved efficiency of the diaphragm muscle. Also, by positioning the hands or arms so that they are supported, the shoulders are stabilized, allowing the neck muscles (called accessory muscles of breathing) to contribute to inhaling air into the lungs.

MUSIC

The soothing power of music is well known. It has a unique link to our emotions and can be helpful in reducing feelings of stress. Listening to music can have a relaxing effect on the brain and affects the body by slowing the heart rate and breathing rate. Studies show that music can act as a distraction that reduces perceived exertion (how difficult it feels) and shortness of breath (how hard it is to breathe) during exercise.

Musical preference varies among individuals. So, you can decide what type of music that you like and what is relaxing. It may also be helpful to listen to different types of music for variety. For example, you may discover that classical music may be calming. Singing along with the music can release tension. Listening to music while exercising can take away feelings that the activity is hard or boring.

PURSED-LIPS BREATHING

This technique is described in chapter 1 ("How to Breathe").

Treatments for Those with Specific Conditions

This information applies to those who have specific conditions that contribute to shortness of breath. Table 9.1 provides an overview of these conditions and individualized therapies.

INSPIRATORY MUSCLE TRAINING

Chapter 1 describes information about the respiratory muscles. In brief, the diaphragm is the main muscle used to breathe in air. Intercostal muscles that connect ribs as well as neck muscles

Table 9.1 Specific conditions

CONDITION		INDIVIDUALIZED THERAPIES
Weak inspiratory muscles	→	Inspiratory muscle training
Exercise limitation and deconditioning	→	Exercise training with assistance
		Noninvasive ventilatory support
		Neuromuscular electrical stimulation
Large bulla	→	Bullectomy
Upper-lobe emphysema	→	Volume-reduction surgery
A benign or malignant growth blocking a breathing tube	→	Laser therapy or stent placement

can assist the diaphragm. Weakness of these inspiratory muscles may develop as a result of

an upper respiratory tract infection;
thyroid disease;
a nerve injury (phrenic nerve) that affects the breathing muscles;
general muscle weakness associated with deconditioning or a
     neuromuscular disease;
COPD; or
congestive heart failure.

Weak inspiratory muscles make it hard or difficult to breathe at rest, with daily activities, and when lying on your back.

Simple breathing tests called *mouth pressures* can be performed to test the strength of the breathing muscles. Low inspiratory and expiratory mouth pressures indicate that the breathing muscles are weak. Handheld devices with adjustable resistances are available for training at home. Different studies show that strengthening the inspiratory muscles improves shortness of breath. Usual training recommendations are as follows:

frequency: at least five days per week

intensity: at least 30 percent of your maximal inspiratory muscle
pressure

duration: usually fifteen minutes twice a day

EXERCISE TRAINING WITH
NONINVASIVE VENTILATION

Noninvasive ventilation (NIV) refers to a breathing machine
that delivers air through tubing into a mask that covers the nose,
mouth, or both, and then into the lungs. An example of the tubing
and mask is shown in figure 9.2. There has been an increasing interest in the use of NIV to reduce breathlessness.

The assisted ventilation reduces the work of the breathing
muscles and allows individuals to train at higher levels of exercise
intensity. NIV could be used as part of a pulmonary rehabilitation
program for selected individuals. At the present time, NIV has
been tried mainly in those with COPD.

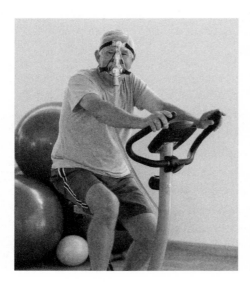

Figure 9.2 Plastic
mask that covers the
nose and mouth is
connected by tubing to
a breathing machine
(ventilator). When the
person starts to breathe
in, the machine delivers
air through the tubing
into the lungs. This should
make it easier to breathe
and enable a person to
do more exercise.
(Based on iStock.com
images from Wavebreak
and John_Brueske)

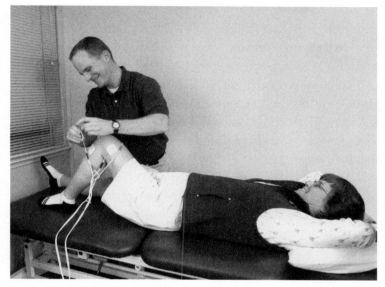

Figure 9.3 Neuromuscular electrical stimulation is done by passing an electrical impulse from a device through electrodes placed on the skin over the targeted muscles. (iStock.com/leezsnow)

NEUROMUSCULAR ELECTRICAL STIMULATION

Some individuals with advanced heart and lung disease are too weak and therefore unable to participate in an exercise program. Neuromuscular electrical stimulation is used alone or combined with a rehabilitation program to strengthen muscles by providing an electrical current through electrodes on the skin over the weak muscle. An example is shown in figure 9.3. The electrical current makes the muscle contract or tighten and get stronger over time. This technique has the potential to allow those with chronic heart or lung disease who have weak muscles to increase strength, then increase physical activities, and then participate in a cardiac or pulmonary rehabilitation program. This process should eventually improve the troubling symptom of breathlessness.

BULLECTOMY

A bulla is an air-filled space at least one centimeter (just less than half an inch) in size (diameter) in the lung. A giant bulla occupies at least 30 percent of one side of the chest. The most common cause of lung bulla is COPD. Other conditions include alpha-1 antitrypsin deficiency (a hereditary form of emphysema), sarcoidosis, smoking cocaine, and intravenous drug use. A bulla may also develop as a result of pneumonia or may occur without a specific cause.

A bulla can compress adjacent normal lung tissue and exert pressure on the diaphragm. Over time, bullae generally get larger and cause more shortness of breath. However, the rate of expansion is unpredictable. The main symptoms are severe breathlessness, repeated infection, and coughing up blood.

Surgical removal of a large bulla (called a bullectomy) deflates the lung and also enables the compressed lung to reexpand. As a result, the diaphragm muscle can lengthen and become more efficient, making it easier to breathe. The operation can be performed in those who have

severe shortness of breath;
a single bulla that occupies at least one-third of one side of the chest; and
evidence on CT scan of the chest that the bulla is compressing the adjacent lung.

Studies suggest that improvements can last for five or more years in 60–90 percent of individuals.

LUNG VOLUME-REDUCTION SURGERY

This is a surgical procedure in which 20–30 percent of tissue in the upper lung zones is removed, usually by video-assisted thoracic surgery (VATS). Figure 9.4 shows a simple illustration of VATS. The goal is to remove emphysema tissue that is not work-

Figure 9.4 Illustration of video-assisted thoracic surgery (VATS) on one side of the chest. Three small incisions are made in different spaces between ribs. A camera is placed into one opening; a clip is placed into another opening; and a biopsy forcep is placed into a third opening. (Based on iStock.com images from elenabs and kowalska-art)

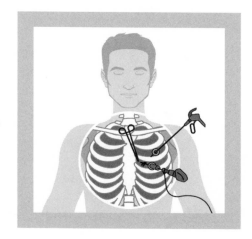

ing and is also pushing the diaphragm down (similar effect as a lung bulla).

The results of the National Emphysema Treatment Trial described the benefits of lung volume-reduction surgery compared with continued medical therapy in 1,212 individuals with severe emphysema. The overall findings were that those with emphysema mainly in the upper areas of the lung and a low exercise capacity benefited from lung volume-reduction surgery with less shortness of breath and better quality of life. Extensive testing is required if you have the emphysema type of COPD in order to determine whether you will likely benefit. In the United States, thoracic surgeons at certain health-care centers perform this procedure.

BRONCHOSCOPIC VOLUME REDUCTION

This procedure was introduced as a less invasive approach to reduce breathlessness in those with advanced emphysema. The goal is the same as for lung volume-reduction surgery: to reduce hyperinflated areas of the lung and thereby improve the function

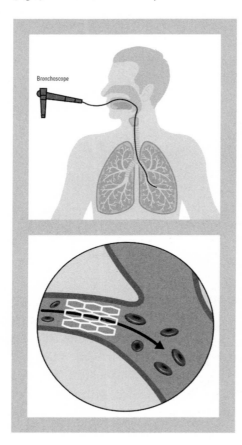

Figure 9.5 Diagram of a bronchoscope placed into the mouth and advanced through the vocal cords into the windpipe and breathing tubes. (Based on iStock.com images from elenabs and kowalska-art)

Figure 9.6 Example of a one-way valve placed into a breathing tube leading to an area of emphysema in the lung. Air (represented by round disks) can only move out of the lung, resulting in collapse of the lung. (iStock.com/stock_shoppe)

of the diaphragm muscle to reduce shortness of breath. The technique involves placing a flexible scope into the mouth and passing it between the vocal cords into the windpipe (trachea) and breathing tubes (airways). This is called a *bronchoscopy* (see figure 9.5). Then, a plastic catheter or tube is placed through a channel in the scope that has a one-way valve or coil at the end. The valve is positioned into a breathing tube leading to an emphysema area of the lung. The valve allows air to move out of the lung but not to

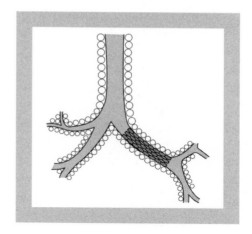

Figure 9.7 Stent is placed into left main breathing tube (called left main stem bronchus) to keep it open and prevent a tumor from blocking airflow. (LeftRightCreative)

enter it. This is shown in figure 9.6. With the removal of air, the area of the lung collapses and deflates the lung.

At the present time, bronchoscopic volume reduction is only available as part of a research program in the United States. However, it is widely used in Europe to treat advanced emphysema.

LASER THERAPY AND STENT PLACEMENT

Tumors (both benign and malignant) can grow in a breathing tube (airway) and block airflow causing breathing difficulty. Laser therapy can be used to destroy the growth and allow air to flow in and out. Also, a stent can be placed into the breathing tube to keep it open as shown in figure 9.7.

Acupuncture: An Emerging Therapy

According to traditional Chinese medicine, *qi* is the fundamental life energy of the universe. It is invisible and found in air, water, food, and sunlight. In the body, it is the vital force that creates and animates life. Each person is born with inherited amounts of *qi*, and it can be obtained from food and the air that you breathe. The

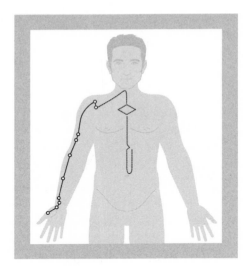

Figure 9.8 The lung meridian route begins in the upper abdomen, moves down to meet the large intestine, moves up and crosses the diaphragm, and then divides and enters the lungs. It then passes up the windpipe, over the shoulder, and down the front of the arm to the wrist and hand. (Based on iStock.com images from elenabs and kowalska-art)

level and quality of your *qi* depends on the state of physical, mental, and emotional balance.

Bodily functions are regulated by *qi* that flows from inside the body to the skin, muscles, tendons, bones, and joints by channels called *meridians*. Disruptions of this flow are believed to be responsible for symptoms and disease. Based on this premise, shortness of breath is due to a deficiency in the flow of *qi* in the lungs. Figure 9.8 shows the lung meridian route.

Acupuncture is a family of procedures that aim to correct the imbalances in the flow of *qi* by stimulation of locations on or under the skin. The most common technique is placement of thin metal needles that penetrate the skin. The depth of insertion of needles varies, depending on which *qi* channels are being treated. Some points barely go beyond superficial layers of skin, while some acupuncture points require a depth of one to three inches of the needle. Although the needles do not generally cause pain, some individuals may report a pinching sensation. Depending on the medical problem, the acupuncturist might spin or move the needles, or even pass a slight electrical current through some of the needles. How long the needles stay inserted into the skin varies. For some individuals, only a quick "in and out" insertion to clear a problem is performed. Other conditions might require that needles remain inserted for up to an hour or more. A related but different approach is to place electrode pads over the acupuncture points and then apply electrical stimulation. This is commonly called transcutaneous electrical nerve stimulation (TENS).

There are ten acupuncture points for the lung meridian as listed in table 9.2. The corresponding acupuncture sites are shown in figure 9.9.

Based on traditional Chinese medicine, stimulating these points can help to relieve various symptoms. At the present time, six studies have compared acupuncture or TENS over acupuncture points with a sham (or pretend) treatment in a total of 256 individuals with COPD. In five of the six studies, there was improvement in shortness of breath with acupuncture therapy or TENS compared with the sham or pretend treatment. One possible reason that acupuncture relieves shortness of breath is the release of endorphins into the fluid around the brain (cerebrospinal fluid).

Key Points

> Some individuals with chronic heart or lung disease remain short of breath despite best available treatments.
> Other strategies for relief of shortness of breath should be considered for these individuals.
> Simple and inexpensive strategies are as follows:
    1 Air movement using a fan
    2 Leaning forward position
    3 Music
    4 Pursed-lips breathing
    5 Triggers that promote release of endorphins

Table 9.2 Acupuncture points for the lung meridian

CHINESE NAME	ENGLISH TRANSLATION	INDICATIONS*
LU-1 Zhong Fu	Central Palace	chest pain; cough; dyspnea; wheezing
LU-2 Yun Men	Cloud Door	cough
LU-3 Tian Fu	Heavenly Residence	cough; psychological issues
LU-4 Xia Bai	Guarding White	cough; dyspnea
LU-5 ChiZe	Cubit Marsh	cough; dyspnea; wheezing
LU-6 Kong Zui	Maximum Opening	chest pain; cough; coughing up blood
LU-7 Lie Que	Broken Sequence	cough
LU-8 Jing Qu	Channel Canal	chest pain; cough; dyspnea
LU-9 Tai Yuan	Great Abyss	chest pain; cough; coughing up blood; dyspnea
LU-10 Yu Ji	Fish Border	chest pain; cough; dyspnea

*There are other indications for each of the points; only respiratory symptoms are listed.
Dyspnea is the medical word for shortness of breath.

> Specific therapies are available based on individual conditions (see table 9.1).
> Acupuncture is an emerging therapy based on positive results in five studies of those with COPD.

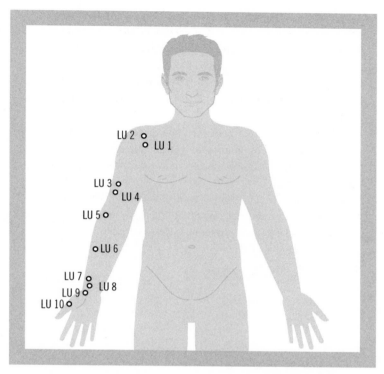

Figure 9.9 LU-1 to LU-10 acupuncture sites. (Based on iStock.com images from elenabs and kowalska-art)

References

Ambrosino, Nicolino, and Paolo Cigni. "Noninvasive Ventilation as an Additional Tool for Exercise Training." *Multidisciplinary Respiratory Medicine* 10 (2015): 1–6.

Galbraith, Sarah, et al. "Does the Use of a Handheld Fan Improve Chronic Dyspnea? A Randomized, Controlled, Crossover Trial." *Journal of Pain and Symptom Management* 39 (2010): 831–38.

Klooster, Karin, et al. "Endobronchial Valves for Emphysema without Interlobar Collateral Ventilation." *New England Journal of Medicine* 373 (2015): 2325–35.

Mahler, Donald A. "Other Treatments for Dyspnea." In *Dyspnea: Mechanisms, Measurement, and Management*, edited by Donald A. Mahler and Denis E. O'Donnell, 207–21. 3rd ed. Boca Raton, FL: CRC Press, 2014.

———. "A Perspective on Acupuncture Techniques for Relief of Dyspnea in Chronic Obstructive Pulmonary Disease." *Medical Acupuncture* 28 (2016): 28–32.

National Emphysema Treatment Trial Research Group. "A Randomized Trial Comparing Lung-Volume-Reduction Surgery with Medical Therapy for Severe Emphysema." *New England Journal of Medicine* 348 (2003): 2059–73.

O'Donnell, Denis E., et al. "Mechanisms of Relief of Exertional Breathlessness following Unilateral Bullectomy and Lung Volume Reduction Surgery in Emphysema." *Chest* 110 (1996): 18–27.

(10)

Traveling with Oxygen

The air up there in the clouds is very pure and fine,
bracing and delicious. And why shouldn't it be? — it is
the same as the angels breathe.

Mark Twain, author and humorist (1835–1910)

Have you been invited to a special event somewhere such as a family wedding, birthday celebration, or school reunion? Do you want to travel to somewhere warmer in the winter months? These opportunities for enjoyment and pleasure may also raise concerns about travel. This chapter discusses the use of oxygen in a personal vehicle, when using public transportation such as on a bus or train, and when traveling by air. Although these situations may be a challenge, planning and preparation should make travel easier and hopefully less stressful.

Supplemental oxygen is available in tanks (cylinders) and in concentrators. An oxygen concentrator is a machine that concentrates the oxygen from air by removing nitrogen. There are both stationary and portable oxygen concentrators (POCs). A POC provides greater flexibility than using oxygen tanks when traveling (figure 10.1). For example, you will not have to worry about switching to another cylinder tank when the one that you are using runs out of oxygen. Also, you will be able to leave the cruise ship when it docks to see local sites without carrying multiple oxygen tanks. Some durable medical equipment companies allow you to rent a POC for travel at a modest cost. Make sure to carry a copy of your oxygen prescription from your health-care provider at all times.

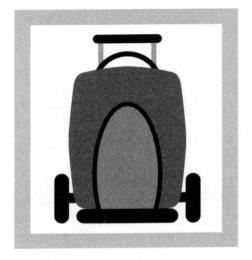

Figure 10.1 Example of a portable oxygen concentrator. (LeftRightCreative)

Traveling by Personal Vehicle

One of the most important things when traveling by car, truck, or motor home is proper storage of your oxygen supply. Tanks should be strapped down behind the front seats in the vehicle. They can be placed on the back seat only if they are fully secured from movement when the vehicle is moving. The oxygen should never be stored in the trunk.

The same information applies if you are using a POC. The POC can be placed on the floor or on the passenger seat if secured. A DC power adapter can be plugged into a power supply in order to charge batteries. This is similar to using a cell-phone car charger. Some guidelines for traveling with oxygen in a personal vehicle are as follows:

While using oxygen, never smoke or be near anyone who is smoking.

Never store or leave oxygen tanks or concentrator in a hot car.

Do not store anything on top of a portable oxygen concentrator.

Store and secure oxygen equipment in an upright position.

Do not store oxygen tanks in the trunk.

Keep windows partially open to prevent oxygen from building up in the vehicle.

Keep the phone number of the company that supplies your oxygen to you.

Traveling by Bus

Travel using a commercial bus line such as Greyhound is fairly easy. Greyhound requires a call forty-eight hours before travel. To notify Greyhound or to arrange assistance, call the Customers with Disabilities phone line at 1-800-752-4841. Companies often require that you show your oxygen prescription and have a doctor's note to travel. Make sure to find out this information from the company and obtain these documents from your health-care provider.

Oxygen tanks and POCs are allowed on buses. However, each bus company will have their own policies and procedures for traveling with oxygen. Greyhound allows you to take four oxygen tanks with you. You can take two tanks aboard the bus with you, while two tanks will remain in the cargo compartments as checked baggage. The maximum dimension for each container is four and a half inches in diameter and twenty-six inches in length. Those stored in the baggage compartment must be in protective cases with safety caps on the valves.

Traveling by Train

Amtrak requires at least twelve hours advance notice if you are traveling with a portable oxygen system. The general Amtrak phone number is 1-800-872-7245. You will then be prompted to respond to various options. You should indicate "special needs" and should then be connected to a representative who can assist you.

The total allowed weight of all oxygen cylinders is 120 pounds. Amtrak allows up to two tanks weighing fifty pounds each or up to six tanks weighing twenty pounds or less each. Because of the planning required and challenge of transporting oxygen tanks, it makes sense to use a POC if possible. The POC must be able to operate with lithium-ion batteries for a minimum of four hours. If you book a first class, business class, or sleeper car, you will likely have access to a standard 110-volt outlet to power your POC.

Traveling by Sea

The cruise industry has welcomed those traveling with oxygen for years. It is important to contact the cruise line to find out about its policies and procedures. They will likely require that you show your oxygen prescription and a doctor's note to travel.

Traveling by Air

As air travel is common, opportunities have increased for those with serious medical conditions to attend an event or vacation somewhere beyond a distance for driving.

If you have a chronic lung condition, you should see your healthcare provider to discuss the following important questions:

Can I fly safely?
Will I need oxygen during the flight?
Where do I get oxygen for air travel?

To answer these questions, it is important to understand the changes that occur when cruising at an altitude of thirty thousand feet in an airplane compared with living at sea level. If you are healthy, you don't even need to think about these issues. However,

Figure 10.2 This figure shows that atmospheric pressure (the weight of air on the earth is shown on the axis on the left) falls as altitude increases (axis at the bottom). (LeftRightCreative)

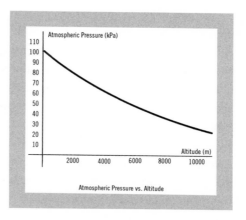

if you have a chronic lung condition, you want to make sure that air travel is safe and uneventful. You will also want to be prepared for any medical problem that could develop.

Medical emergencies during air travel are uncommon. In one study it was estimated that there was one medical emergency for every six hundred flights. About 12 percent of these in-air emergencies were for respiratory complaints. Other emergencies include passing out, heart problems, and strokes.

WHAT HAPPENS TO THE OXYGEN LEVEL IN INHALED AIR DURING AIR TRAVEL?

This section provides a brief and hopefully simple explanation about the changes inside the airplane (called the aircraft cabin) when flying. As the airplane climbs, the pressure inside the cabin falls as shown in figure 10.2. Most commercial airplanes fly at a cruising altitude of thirty to forty thousand feet above sea level. The Federal Aviation Administration requires that pressure inside the airplane (called the cabin pressure) be maintained at an altitude of about eight thousand feet above sea level under normal operating conditions.

To pressurize the airplane, up to 50 percent of the air in the cabin is expelled from the plane and is replaced by air outside the airplane (exterior air). This exterior air is compressed and then mixed with filtered and recirculated air in the cabin. There are about twenty to thirty complete air exchanges per hour. As the airplane climbs, the decrease in cabin pressure results in gas expansion that can cause a "popping" sensation in the ears of passengers.

With reduced pressure in the cabin, there is reduced oxygen in the air. At normal flying altitude (cabin pressure equal to eight thousand feet above sea level), the oxygen in the air is 15 percent compared with 21 percent at sea level. Healthy passengers can tolerate this reduction in inspired oxygen without any breathing difficulty or medical problem. However, in an effort to compensate for the lower oxygen in the air (15 percent), someone with a chronic lung condition responds by breathing more and with a faster heart rate. This may lead to breathing difficulty.

Various medical conditions increase the risk of possible problems as a result of the low oxygen in the cabin of the airplane. In those with asthma and chronic obstructive pulminary disease (COPD), the increase in breathing may result in air being trapped in the lungs causing it to overinflate. This makes shortness of breath worse. Those with interstitial lung disease, kyphoscoliosis (curvature of the spine), and obesity may be limited in their ability to increase breathing. Heart disease, sleep apnea, pulmonary hypertension, and cystic fibrosis may also contribute to possible in-flight problems.

WILL YOU NEED OXYGEN?

If you have a chronic lung condition, a preflight screening is recommended. This evaluation includes a medical history, physical examination, and breathing tests. You may wish to ask your primary care provider if he or she performs such evaluations. If not, then you should schedule an appointment with a lung specialist (pulmonologist). At the medical visit, any previous flying experience as well as any problems during air travel should be discussed. Oxygen saturation (SpO2) should be measured by pulse oximetry while breathing room air. If your SpO2 is 95 percent or higher, then no testing is necessary. If your SpO2 is below 95 percent, then additional testing is recommended.

Hypoxic (this is a medical word that means a low oxygen level) challenge is a special breathing test to assess the risk of a low oxygen level when flying. With this test, you breathe 15 percent oxygen for twenty minutes to simulate the conditions when flying at a cabin pressure of eight thousand feet. If the SpO2 is less than 85 percent during the hypoxic challenge test, then oxygen is recommended during air travel. The recommended flow rate is two liters per minute. The hypoxic challenge test is usually available at medical centers, large hospitals, and possibly some community hospitals. If the SpO2 is 85 percent or higher, then oxygen is not needed for air travel.

If you are already using oxygen therapy 24-7, then the flow rate should be increased by two liters per minute for air travel. As an example, if you are using oxygen at two liters per minute at rest, then the flow rate should be increased to four liters per minute during air travel.

Recommendations for hypoxic testing and need for oxygen are summarized in table 10.1.

HOW TO ARRANGE FOR OXYGEN
DURING AIR TRAVEL

The process of arranging for oxygen to use during air travel can be challenging. As the passenger, you are responsible for making arrangements with the specific airline. All airlines require that the traveler make the request for oxygen *in advance* and require that a health-care provider complete a form documenting the diagnosis

Table 10.1 Summary of recommendations for using oxygen
during air travel

OXYGEN SATURATION AT REST AT SEA LEVEL	HYPOXIC CHALLENGE TEST	NEED FOR OXYGEN
95% or higher	No	No
Below 95%	Yes	Yes, if SpO2 is less than 85% during test. Use oxygen at 2 liters/minute.
Currently using oxygen 24-7	No	Increase usual flow rate by 2 liters/minute.

and need for oxygen as well as the specific flow rate. How oxygen is
provided for an individual traveler depends, in part, on the policy
of the airline. There are two options for using oxygen while flying
in the airplane:

1 The airline can provide the oxygen.

   OR

2 You can provide the oxygen by using a POC.

Airlines will arrange for use of supplemental oxygen according to their policies. The Airline Oxygen Council of America has a
website that lists these policies for in-flight oxygen use and equipment (www.airlineoxygencouncil.org). You will need to inform
the airline when you make a reservation that you will need oxygen
during the flight. Federal regulations prohibit airlines from allowing passengers to bring their own oxygen tanks on the airplane.
Some key questions to ask the airline personnel are listed below:

Does the airline accept passengers who require oxygen?
Is oxygen supplied by the airline, or can I bring my POC on
    the flight?

How much time is required (days or weeks) for notification
    before the flight?

What kind of note is required by my health-care provider?
    (Most if not all airlines require a signed copy of your oxygen
    prescription as well as a written statement from your health-
    care provider.)

Does the airline select specific seats for those traveling with
    oxygen?

How much will it cost if I use oxygen provided by the airline
    during the flight? (The charge may be $100 to $250 per flight
    depending on the flight travel time.)

Does the airline supply nasal cannula or a face mask for use with
    oxygen? Or should I bring my own tubing system?

Since 2009, all airlines traveling to and from the United States
are required by law to permit passengers to carry their own POC as
long as the individual has been approved to use oxygen while flying. The system must be a Federal Aviation Agency (FAA) approved
oxygen concentrator. Remember, the POC removes nitrogen from
the air (air contains 21 percent oxygen and 79 percent nitrogen)
and can deliver a higher concentration of oxygen.

Individuals must typically provide at least forty-eight hours' notice of your plan to travel along with a doctor's statement about
how and when the POC is to be used during the flight. If you are
not currently using a POC, consider a short-term rental from an
oxygen supply company because a POC is easier for the traveler,
especially if oxygen is needed before and after flying. Because
airlines may not provide a power outlet for using a POC, the system should be fully charged. Also, you will need to bring enough
twelve-cell batteries for one and half times the anticipated duration of the flight. For example, if your flight is four hours, you will
need six hours of battery life. While at the airport, you will likely be
able to plug the POC into an electrical outlet to save power.

If you are currently using oxygen, it is important to contact the company that supplies your oxygen to ask what services, if any, that it provides before and after the flight. You should discuss with an employee of the company how to make sure that oxygen is available at the airport before the departing flight; at the airport upon arrival and where you are staying; and at the airport before your return flight.

You will need to inform the oxygen supply company of the flight numbers along with departure and arrival times. Make sure to have the local phone number of the company and a contact person in case of any unforeseen situation. Using a POC for air travel is convenient and eliminates many of the above concerns.

WHAT TO DO ON THE PLANE BEFORE TAKEOFF

After you board the plane and before it leaves the gate, you should make sure that

the oxygen equipment is working properly;
you have easy access to the batteries if needed for the POC;
the flow meter is set at the correct rate; and
inhalers are available if needed.

WHO SHOULD NOT FLY?

Anyone with a communicable disease such as tuberculosis should not fly in a commercial airplane. Also, anyone with an unresolved pneumothorax (rupture of air into space around the lungs) should not fly because air trapped in the pleural space will expand at altitude. Most airlines will accept someone who recently had chest (thoracic) surgery after two weeks of recovery, but assessment by a health-care provider is important.

Figure 10.3 On the right is shown a blood clot inside a vein. On the left is shown the location of the blood clot just above the left knee. (Based on iStock.com images from elenabs, kowalska-art, and stock_shoppe)

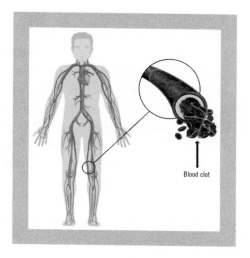

Blood clot

A Risk of Prolonged Travel: Venous Thromboembolism

Venous thromboembolism means blood clots in the veins of the legs (figure 10.3). Part or all of the clot may break away and travel to the lungs (called pulmonary embolism). If this occurs, you may experience sudden shortness of breath and chest pain. Sitting for a long time in the seat and dehydration are contributing factors to the risk of venous thromboembolism. Low oxygen in the air of the cabin pressured for eight thousand feet does not contribute to the formation of blood clots. It is important to get out of your seat often during travel (personal vehicle, bus, train, and plane) to walk around and stretch to reduce the risk of blood clots developing.

Traveling to a High Altitude

Oxygen levels in the air are reduced at a high altitude. For example, at Denver, which is 5,280 feet above sea level, there is 18 percent oxygen in the air compared with 21 percent at sea level. Your body adjusts for the lower oxygen by breathing more frequently and by a faster heart rate. Whether you notice these changes depends on each person and the severity of any chronic lung or heart condition.

Compared with usual physical activities that you perform at home, these same tasks may make you feel short of breath and more tired at high altitude. Staying overnight at a high altitude will likely affect your sleep. Poor sleep quality may cause common complaints such as not being able to sleep and being awake at night. If possible, you may consider traveling to higher elevations in stages to minimize problems. For example, you may wish to stay overnight in Denver for one to two nights before traveling to a higher altitude in the Rocky Mountains.

If you have a chronic lung condition and are not using oxygen where you live, you should ask your health-care provider whether oxygen is necessary at a high altitude. Other general recommendations are to limit physical activities for a few days, drink plenty of water, and avoid alcohol. Having an action plan in case of breathing difficulties is also important.

Disease-Specific Recommendations

Certain respiratory conditions might affect air travel. If you have any of these diseases, make sure to discuss any health concerns with your health-care provider before traveling.

ASTHMA

Commercial air travel does not pose a problem in those with asthma. Certainly, you want to have your asthma under good control before flying. Make sure to carry all inhalers as well as any pills that you take for asthma on the plane. In particular, you should have a rescue albuterol inhaler and prednisone available in case of an emergency.

COPD

The frequency of severe air-travel-related problems is low in those with COPD. As with asthma, it is important to carry all of your inhalers on the plane for two reasons: you might need your rescue albuterol or maintenance medications; and you want to be sure that you have medications when you arrive at your destination and not take a chance that your luggage could be lost.

Those with COPD are at risk for expansion of any closed air pockets such as a lung bulla during air travel. Because of changes in pressure in the airplane, the air within the bulla can expand and possibly rupture. Your health-care provider can let you know if you have a lung bulla based on a chest x-ray or CT scan of the chest.

INTERSTITIAL LUNG DISEASE

Those with interstitial lung disease should see a lung specialist (pulmonologist) before air travel to assess for the need for oxygen and for emergency supplies of antibiotics and prednisone.

UPPER RESPIRATORY TRACT INFECTION

If you have a viral upper respiratory tract infection, commonly called a "cold," you may experience ear pain or congestion, especially when the plane descends. Either nasal or oral decongestants may help with symptoms if taken before air travel.

If you are coughing, it is advisable that you wear a mask to cover your nose and mouth.

PNEUMONIA

If you have pneumonia, you should ask your health-care provider if it is safe to fly. Common sense suggests that you should only travel if your temperature is normal; you are feeling close to your normal self; and the pneumonia has been adequately treated to minimize transmission to other passengers.

If you are coughing, it is advisable that you wear a mask to cover your nose and mouth.

OBSTRUCTIVE SLEEP APNEA

A doctor's letter is required outlining the diagnosis and the necessary equipment (mask and positive airway pressure machine) that will need to be carried on the plane. A useful fact sheet is available on the Internet at www.sleepapnea.org.

Key Points

> In a commercial airplane flying at cruising altitude (about thirty thousand feet above sea level), the concentration of oxygen in the air is 15 percent compared to 21 percent at sea level.

> Healthy individuals and most of those with a chronic lung condition can tolerate this reduced oxygen in inspired air without any problem.

> If you have a chronic respiratory condition, you should see a health-care provider to discuss the following important questions:

  1 Can I fly safely?

  2 Will I need oxygen during the flight?

  3 Where do I get oxygen for air travel?

> Neither breathing tests nor measuring oxygen saturation at sea level can predict whether an individual with a chronic heart or lung condition will experience a low oxygen level during air travel.

> A special breathing test called hypoxic challenge may be used to simulate the conditions in the airplane to determine whether you will need oxygen during air travel.

> Traveling with oxygen requires planning and preparation. It is important to inform the travel company in advance

of your need to use oxygen and to carry the written oxygen prescription and a note from your health-care provider with you.

> A portable oxygen concentrator (POC) provides greater flexibility and ease compared with using oxygen tanks for travel.

> Most airlines can provide oxygen at two to four liters per minute flow rate with advance notice if oxygen is necessary for air travel.

> Make sure to carry your inhalers and other medicines with you on the flight.

References

Josephs, Lynn K., Robina K. Coker, and Mike Thomas. "Managing Patients with Stable Respiratory Disease Planning Air Travel: A Primary Care Summary of the British Thoracic Society Recommendations." *Primary Care Respiratory Journal* 22 (2013): 234–38.

Nicholson, Trevor T., and Jacob I. Sznajder. "Fitness to Fly in Patients with Lung Disease." *Annals of the American Thoracic Society* 11 (2014): 1614–22.

Robson, A. G., and J. A. Innes. "Problems of Air Travel for Patients with Lung Disease: Clinical Criteria and Regulations." *Breathe* 3 (2006): 141–47.

Stoller, James K. "Patient Information: Supplemental Oxygen on Commercial Airlines (Beyond the Basics)." UpToDate. Last updated June 30, 2015. http://www.uptodate.com/.

Index

Page references in *italics* refer to figures and tables.